MIND
HEALING

MIND HEALING

Ten Lectures by TCM Experts

EDITOR-IN-CHIEF
ZHU HUIRONG

DEPUTY EDITORS
CHENG LIN   TAO SILIANG

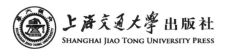
上海交通大學出版社
SHANGHAI JIAO TONG UNIVERSITY PRESS

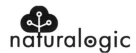
naturalogic

Mind Healing:
Ten Lectures by TCM Experts

Editor-in-Chief: Zhu Huirong
Deputy editors: Cheng Lin & Tao Siliang

Copyright © Shanghai Jiao Tong University Press

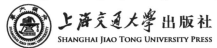

上海交通大学出版社
SHANGHAI JIAO TONG UNIVERSITY PRESS

Published by NATURALOGIC PUBLISHING INC., under an exclusive license with Shanghai Jiao Tong University Press.

First English Edition 2022
ISBN: 978-1-4878-0904-1

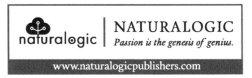

naturalogic | NATURALOGIC
Passion is the genesis of genius.
www.naturalogicpublishers.com

19-1235 Johnson St. Coquitlam, BC, Canada V3B 7E2

Foreword

In recent years, increasing scholars learned from the wisdom of advantages of traditional Chinese medicine. The way traditional Chinese medicine understands psychology and treats mental illness is different from that of Western medicine, psychiatry and psychology. TCM theories embody the survival wisdom and cultural characteristics of the Chinese nation, and TCM treatments are simple, convenient, economical and effective. *The Inner Canon of the Yellow Emperor* (*Huáng Dì Nèi Jīng*, 黄帝内经), the earliest Chinese medical classic, is rich in ideas of psychosomatic medicine and psychology. It involves topics in modern psychology. Now, there are well-organized theories of TCM psychology with characteristics of Chinese culture and many effective emotion focused therapies. Professor Wang Qingqi in Shanghai University of Traditional Chinese Medicine encouraged students in TCM Psychology Master Studio to learn more experience, and demonstrated how to spread TCM culture and combine TCM with psychology.

It is common sense in TCM to distinguish between cold and heat, differentiate Yin from Yang, and balance deficiency and excess, for patients suffering from physical diseases. The same is true of patients with mental illness. We can help patients actively heal themselves with education and emotion focus therapies by strengthening healthy qi to balance Yin and Yang, and improving physical and mental immunity, if we take mental disorders seriously as diseases and apply the TCM idea of "primarily treating patients with illness but not diseases affecting people" to psychology. For patients troubled by mental illness, we can also differentiate deficiency from excess, and distinguish healthy qi from evil qi, based on which treatments can be given to strengthen healthy qi and expel evil qi so as to balance Yin and Yang and restore health, according to specific body constitutions of patients.

Zhu Huirong is my student. As a brilliant oncologist in traditional Chinese medicine, she has been caring about mental health of patients. Since several years ago, she has been interested in the research achievements of psychologists in China. In recent years, she has tried to offer services of TCM psychology to college students. She not only did it by herself or with a team, but also invited many experts to work jointly. I really appreciate that.

This book includes the speeches by Wang Qingqi, He Yumin, Qu Lifang and Li Zhaojian in Shanghai University of Traditional Chinese Medicine. It also contains academic achievements of outstanding experts including Wang Keqin from Heilongjiang, Yang Qiuli from Beijing, and Zhang Bohua from Shandong. Their insights gather in this one book. I believe this book will bring readers closer to traditional Chinese culture, inspire them with energy, and help them better understand the meaning of life from a Chinese perspective. On this basis, it is of epoch-making significance if the theories and technologies of TCM psychology can be used creatively and properly to maintain and improve mental health.

I hope that this book can enlighten TCM scholars, psychologists and educators and become an important reference for all readers who attach importance to traditional Chinese culture. I wish Shanghai University of Traditional Chinese Medicine make greater achievements in TCM mental health education and make greater contributions to the world.

LIU JIAXIANG

February 2018

Entitled to special government allowances from the State Council in China, Liu Jiaxiang is a master of traditional Chinese medicine, a tenured professor in Shanghai University of Traditional Chinese Medicine, a physician-in-chief and tenured professor in Longhua Hospital affiliated to SHUTCM, a doctoral supervisor, one of the first national postdoctoral supervisors for TCM inheritance, the chief expert in national base of TCM clinical research, the director of National TCM Center for Cancer, the director of Shanghai TCM Center for Cancer, the supervisor for inheritance of academic experience of national TCM famous experts, one of the first Shanghai famous TCM doctors, the vice president of Cancer Specialty Committee of the World Federation of Chinese Medicine Societies, the consultant of Cancer Specialty Committee of the Chinese Association of Integrative Medicine, and the honorary chairman of the cancer branch of the China Association of Chinese medicine.

Preface

On the shores of Saranak Lake in northeast New York, a doctor named Edward Livingston Trudeau has been buried. His widely-known epitaph has inspired generations of medical practitioners. That is "To cure sometimes, To relieve often, To comfort always." The short and concise sentence embodies the core idea of clinical practice, which has encouraged generations of doctors to forge ahead with medical treatment.

As a clinician, I met many patients with tumors and mental disorders. I found that 30% to 50% of patients with advanced malignant tumors had depression, which was often accompanied by anxiety or other symptoms. Years of my clinical experience has made me realize a truth that "mental health contributes to half of overall health, and mental disease contributes to half of overall illness." Therefore, mental health is as important as physical health. The mental state can greatly affect the prognosis and outcome of a disease.

At the same time, as an educator in university, I perceive that mental health education for college students in China should be based on the advantages of traditional Chinese culture, during my experience of moral education. With traditional Chinese medicine as a foundation, we can invent indigenous education model of mental health for college students in China.

Theories of mental health are influenced by cultures. During the development of psychological theories, each had its own historical background, which were put forward for better clinical practice. The same is true of mental health education and counseling. All the theories in Western psychology formed, developed, and improved according to corresponding times and societies. In other words, mental health education and counseling influenced by different cultures have their own characteristics, whose theories and techniques come into being based on the cultures and corresponding backgrounds.

As for the mental health education and counselling for college students in China, theories of Western psychology were commonly used in the past. However, it is not appropriate if we do not modify them for specific situations. Actually, theories of mental health and their techniques in Western universities, such as University of Cambridge and University of Oxford, are keeping pace with practical problems and the development of society.

Therefore, although it is very meaningful to take theories and practical experience of Western psychology as a reference, we should not apply them mechanically in China.

At present, Shanghai University of Traditional Chinese Medicine is trying to construct an indigenous education model of mental health for college students, with the characteristics of TCM culture. We aim to apply theories of TCM psychology to mental health education and counselling for college students.

Through years of exploration, we have been trying to combine Western theories with advantages of traditional Chinese culture and traditional Chinese medicine, in the following three ways.

1. To explore the wisdom of TCM culture for physical and mental health in terms of "philosophy, theory and technology"

The Book of Change (Zhōu Yì, 周易) · Explanations for The Scriptures reads, "those intangible belong to philosophy, while those tangible belong to objects." Ancient Chinese psychology is an inseparable part of traditional Chinese medicine. TCM thought originates from traditional Chinese culture and ancient Chinese philosophy, which has unique epistemological and methodological characteristics. Traditional Chinese medicine advocates the holistic view of "unity of nature and human" and "unity of body and mind." The first chapter of *The Inner Canon of the Yellow Emperor: Basic Questions (Huáng Dì Nèi Jīng Sù Wèn, 黄帝内经素问) · Discourse on the True Qi Endowed by Heaven in High Antiquity* reads that "the people of high antiquity, who understood philosophy, modeled their behavior on yin and yang and complied with the arts and the calculations; their eating and drinking were moderate; their rising and resting had regularity; they did not tax themselves with meaningless work; hence, they were able to keep physical appearance and spirit together, and to exhaust the years allotted by heaven; their life span exceeded one hundred years before they departed."

Basic Questions (Sù Wèn, 素问) · Discourse on How The Generative Qi Communicates with Heaven reads "when yin and yang are balanced and sealed, then essence and spirit are in order." That is to say, with intact body-mind, good physical and mental health, and abundant energy, people can have a longer lifespan. In a sense, traditional Chinese medicine is philosophy of medicine, revealing the art of healing humans physically and mentally. When trying to construct an indigenous education model of mental health for college students, with the characteristics of TCM culture, we aim to find out proper ways of mental health education in terms of philosophy, theory and technology, based on literatures and practice.

2. To reveal the traditional wisdom through "tracing, combining and applying"

"Tracing" is to stick to the philosophy, theory and technology of TCM psychology. "Combining" is to combine TCM psychology with the mainstay of theories in Western psychology. "Applying" is to apply indigenous theories and technologies in practice. We focus on the interpretation of TCM psychology in modern society and aim to explore how to offer services to college students, laying a foundation for better theories and practice of mental health education and counselling for college students in China in the future.

For example, in recent years, we have applied "TCM Rating Scales of Five-Status Personality Test" to the psychological tests for college freshmen. The classification of personalities, body constitutions and physiques in traditional Chinese medicine is discussed in *The Inner Canon of the Yellow Emperor (Huáng Dì Nèi Jīng, 黄帝内经)*, summarized in "five-status classification" and "five-element classification." With "five-status classification," people are divided into five categories based on yin and yang: Greater Yin, Lesser Yin, Greater Yang, Lesser Yang and Balanced Yin-Yang. In *The Inner Canon of the Yellow Emperor (Huáng Dì Nèi Jīng, 黄帝内经)*, behaviors, manners, personalities, body constitutions and treatments are described in detail for five-status classification. The five types of personality have influences on both physical and mental health.

People of Greater Yang are extroverted, emotionally unstable, irritable, ambitious, stubborn, confident, energetic, and aggressive. People of Greater Yin are introverted, emotionally unstable, timid, conservative, sensitive, quiet, indecisive, stubborn, dull, and selfish.

Over the past few years, by comparing the results of TCM Rating Scales of Five-Status Personality Test and the results of SCL-90, it is found that most of the students screened out by SCL-90 belong to people of Greater Yin. There are overlaps between the results, but they are not exactly the same. Therefore, they can supplement each other. There is a significant sign for People of Greater Yin. Studies have shown that Greater Yin correlates with previous suicidal ideation, suicidal ideation in the past year and the possibility of suicide in the future. It also correlates with negative emotions such as depression and loneliness.

It can be considered that Five-Status Personality Test derives from the philosophy of Yin and Yang in traditional Chinese medicine. The philosophy brought out theories. Then, based on scientific methods of psychological scale construction and nationwide test norms, technologies came into being. That is about a whole process of indigenization. Theories form the basis for "tracing." Scientific methods imply "combining." Tests for colleges students are "applying."

3. To construct an effective indigenous model of mental health education and counselling by "understanding, practicing, and evaluating"

"Understanding" is to learn the theories and practical experience of Western psychology and TCM psychology in an unbiased way, according to their corresponding historical and academic backgrounds.

"Practicing" is to apply theories to solving actual problems in the universities in China, on the basis of understanding. "Evaluating" is to determine how theories work in practice. Based on the feedbacks from recipients, evaluations can be conducted to improve the indigenous model of mental health education and counselling.

"Do not forget our original intention, and keep in mind the mission." The report of the 19th National Congress of the Communist Party of China points out that as China is getting closer to the center of the world stage, China's idea, China's wisdom, China's plans, and China's opportunities are increasingly attracting global attention. The new era, new ideas, new mission, and new journey indicate that China has a closer relationship with the world than before. To explore an indigenous model of mental health education and counselling will not only meet the need of China, but also benefit the world in the future.

Generally speaking, what we are doing is still at the very beginning. There are more things that need to be improved and developed. Since the basis is theories, we invited famous experts to our university in the past years to give speeches and compiled this book.

Please let me briefly introduce the lectures involved in this book. Professor Wang Qingqi is a tenured professor in Shanghai University of Traditional Chinese Medicine, with the title of Shanghai Famous TCM Doctor, and the host of TCM Psychology Master Studio. He will interpret the thought of "harmony" in TCM and traditional Chinese culture, explain the connotations and denotations of body and mind, and introduce the role of TCM culture in health preservation. He will also discuss the similarities and differences between stagnation syndrome in TCM and depression in Western medicine, with Professor Wang Zhen who is a physician-in-chief and also the director of teaching department in Shanghai Mental Health Center affiliated to Shanghai Jiao Tong University School of Medicine. Professor He Yumin in Shanghai University of Traditional Chinese Medicine is the director of Chinese Medical Association and former chairman of the psychosomatic medicine branch, who will share his opinions on indigenization of psychology in clinical practice. Professor Wang Keqin in Heilongjiang Academy of Chinese Medical Sciences is the honorary president of TCM psychology specialty committee of World Federation of Chinese Medicine Societies, and an academic leader of TCM psychology. He will introduce the concept of TCM psychology and its basic theories. Professor Qu Lifang in Shanghai University of Traditional Chinese Medicine is the chief editor of *Mental Disorders in TCM (Zhōng Yī Shén Zhì Bìng Xué*, 中医神志病学*)* and *Selected Famous Cases of Psychiatric Disorders of Past Dynasties (Jīng Shén Xīn Lǐ Jí Bìng Lì Dài Míng Jiā Yàn Àn Xuǎn Cuì*, 精神心理疾病历代名家验案选粹*)*. She will elaborate on the relationship between the heart governing the mind and mental development. Yang Qiuli is a scientist in Chinese Academy of Chinese Medical Sciences. She is one of the founders of the first indigenous measure of personality assessment of Five-Status Personality Test and Five-Five Body Constitution Test in China, as well as the standardized measure of mental and physical health assessment in TCM. She will introduce the Body-mind Regulation System of Five-Status. Li Zhaojian is a research fellow in Shanghai University of Traditional Chinese Medicine. He has been engaged in research on psychosomatic medicine since 1995. He will introduce emotion focused therapies of traditional Chinese medicine. Professor Zhang Bohua is the vice president of the specialty committee of TCM psychology of the World Federation of Chinese medicine Societies, a member of the Standing Committee of Chinese Association for Psychological Intervention and president of specialty committee of TCM psychology, an academic leader of TCM psychology, and the founder of psychology discipline in Shandong University of traditional Chinese medicine. She will share her understanding of emotion focused therapies in TCM.

Those experts are not only famous doctors but also good teachers. They have not only broad theoretical vision and rigorous academic attitude, but also profound knowledge of cultures. They have passions for psychology, traditional Chinese medicine, as well as traditional Chinese culture. In their speeches, they not only share academic achievements, but also inherit and spread the advantages of traditional Chinese culture. Their enthusiasm is embodied in every word of this book. TCM psychology can be philosophy, thought, and even a technology. I sincerely hope that this book can give new impetus to the development of TCM psychology, inspire students, health professionals and medical practitioners with new ideas, and arouse people's interest in traditional Chinese culture.

This book integrates the specialties of different experts, discussing theories in both ancient and modern times and involving the philosophy, theory and technology of TCM psychology, with brilliant arguments. If you want to explore more about the opinions in this book after reading, you may refer to monographs by the lectures further.

With the ardent support by the Ministry of education of the People's Republic of China, the Shanghai Municipal Education Commission, and Shanghai Jiao Tong University Press, I would like to express my sincere thanks for the contributions that relevant experts and leaders made to this book. Psychology of traditional Chinese medicine is still a relatively new field. If there are any shortcomings, we would love to receive your opinions.

ZHU HUIRONG

Contents

LECTURE 1

Laying a Foundation

The Scientific Concept and Basic Theoretical Framework of Traditional Chinese Medicine (TCM) Psychology

LECTURER: WANG KEQIN

Introduction to the speaker:

Wang Keqin is a researcher, chief physician, and professor of Heilongjiang Academy of Chinese Medical Sciences. He is also an honorary fellow of Institute of Basic Research in clinical medicine, China Academy of Chinese Medical Sciences, and an honorary chairman of TCM Psychology Professional Committee, WFCMS. As a senior editor of *Yearbook of Traditional Chinese Medicine of China (Academic Volume),* he receives special government allowances of the State Council for his lifetime. During 55 years of study in TCM, Wang has devoted himself to TCM psychology for more than 30 years. He has constructed a "basic theoretical framework of TCM Psychology" and is one of the pioneers in this field.

Traditional Chinese medicine psychology is an interdisciplinary subject of traditional Chinese medicine and psychology. It has a long history because the theoretical origin can be traced back to *The Inner Canon of the Yellow Emperor* or even before. Psychological thoughts abound in the book and many other classics during the pre-Qin period. However, the discipline was established in the early 1980s, and was not recognized by National Administration of Traditional Chinese medicine until the end of 2009. Therefore, TCM psychology is still a brand-new discipline for its acknowledged history of less than 10 years.

1.1 Historical Review on Establishment of TCM Psychology

First of all, I would like to review the history of the discipline establishment with you.

The name of TCM psychology, which is also the earliest concept, was first proposed by Wang Miqu, a professor from Chengdu University of TCM, in the early 1980s. At that time, scientific ideas were just ushered in after the end of Cultural Revolution. Thus, it took courage to put forward the viewpoint in that period. Although I was also studying TCM psychology in the meantime, I only conservatively proposed the theory of Shen in TCM.

In 1985, the birth of the discipline was proclaimed on the first National TCM Psychology Academy Forum in Chengdu, Sichuan. During the meeting, representatives unanimously passed the resolution to develop the subject with concerted efforts. To meet teaching needs for TCM colleges, experts and scholars from 17 colleges and research institutes were organized to compile *Science of Traditional Chinese Medicine Psychology*, among which Wang Miqu, Wang Keqin, Zhu Wenfeng, and Zhang Liutong were appointed as chief editors. The symposium and compilation of the national textbook initiated construction of the emerging discipline. Afterwards a national academic event was held every 1 to 2 years, while academic journals such as *Collected Essays on TCM Psychology* were published. Meanwhile, a national academic organization was in preparation. Through tireless efforts, Research Committee of Traditional Chinese Medicine Psychology, CARDTCM, was established with approval in 1992. Wang Keqin was appointed as the chairman, Du Huaitang, Zhu Wenfeng, and Zhang Liutong as vice-chairmen, and Wang Miqu as the secretary-general. Thus, the first academic organization of TCM psychology was founded.

Then Xue Chongcheng, the grandmaster of TCM psychology, worked hard for official acknowledgement of the discipline. In 2001, National Administration of Traditional Chinese Medicine commissioned China Academy of Chinese Medical Sciences to hold the first feasibility study meeting. In 2006, TCM Psychology

Professional Committee, WFCMS, was established, which introduced TCM psychology to the world. In 2007, the feasibility study meeting of TCM psychology was held again. Finally, in 2009, National Administration of Traditional Chinese Medicine officially recognized TCM psychology as a discipline. Therefore, year 2009 is regarded as a new milestone in the construction and development of TCM psychology.

1.2 Concept of TCM Psychology

Since Wang Miqu first proposed the concept of TCM psychology in the early 1980s, experts and scholars have improved it for decades of years. Now, the concept is basically determined. A few years ago, I was fortunate to serve as an expert advisor in work of "Formulating Term Standards for TCM Psychiatry and Psychology." It is a 2008 national basic research program of science and technology hosted by Yang Qiuli, a professor at China Academy of Chinese Medical Sciences. Gathering suggestions from several experts, the research group standardized terms of TCM psychology and obtained recognition.

First, the project clarified the concept of TCM psychology. "Traditional Chinese Medicine Psychology is a new discipline rooted in traditional Chinese culture. It inherits essence of ancient Chinese psychology and combines research results of modern psychology. Applying theories of traditional Chinese medicine, it interprets psychological phenomena of human beings and explores nature and patterns of psychological activities. Furthermore, the subject studies influence of psychological factors on occurrence, development, and changes of diseases, and thus provides guidance on healthcare, clinical disease prevention and treatment."

Now I will analyze the concept from following aspects.

(1) The concept emphasizes features of TCM psychology. With characteristics of traditional Chinese culture, the discipline inherits essence of ancient Chinese psychology on the basis of TCM theory. TCM psychology is indigenous because it embodies traditional Chinese culture, which is different from western psychology.

(2) The concept summarizes two major research contents of TCM psychology: theoretical research and clinical research.

Theoretical research includes research on history, literature, and basic theory of TCM psychology. *Basic Theory of Traditional Chinese Medicine Psychology*, the textbook Professor Yang Qiuli and I co-authored, was published by People's Medical Publishing House in April, 2013. Theoretical research also includes research on TCM psychopathology, that is, to differentiate causes and mechanisms of mental illness from related TCM theory and improve them with modern psychology research.

Clinical research includes research on TCM psychology diagnosis, measurement, and evaluation. Both four examinations (inspection, listening and smelling, inquiry, and palpation) in TCM and scale questionnaires in western psychology are in use. "Five-Pattern Personality Inventory," a test developed by Grandmaster Xue Chongcheng and Professor Yang Qiuli on the basis of yin-yang theory in *The Inner Canon of the Yellow Emperor*, has filled the gap in localized psychology measurement. Clinical researchers should not only systematically sort out and dig for TCM psychological therapy, but also develop new treatment according to China's domestic conditions, such as Professor Wang Weidong's Thought Imprint Psychotherapy (TIP), and Professor Zhang Bohua's Emotional Homeopathic Psychotherapy. Furthermore, clinical research focuses on application. More research should be conducted on TCM psychological healthcare, TCM psychological nursery, and TCM clinical psychology, especially treatment for some mental diseases such as emotional disorder, mental disease, psychosomatic disease, and sleep disorder. *Clinical Psychology of Traditional Chinese Medicine*, a textbook edited by Professor Zhang Xiaojuan's team, was published by China Medical Science and Technology Press in 2006. It lays foundation for research on TCM clinical psychology.

(3) The concept clarifies that purpose of TCM psychology research is to serve human being's mental and physical health.

1.3   TCM Psychology Inherits Essence of Ancient Chinese Psychology

Rooted in and Embodying traditional Chinese culture, TCM psychology inherits essence of ancient Chinese psychology. Although there was no such discipline as psychology in ancient China, many ancient classics imply precious psychological thoughts. Thus, we worked hard to absorb essence of these ideas when establishing the subject.

(1) "Theory on Preciousness of Man" in Ancient China

Why is man precious? According to ancient classics, preciousness lies in three aspects: judgement, kindness, and aspiration. These three elements exactly correspond to cognition, emotion, and will in psychology. Human beings stand out from other creatures due to distinctive psychological qualities. Thus, theory on preciousness of man emphasizes necessity and importance of psychology research, and basically defines research scope of TCM psychology.

(2) "THEORY ON FORM AND SHEN" IN ANCIENT CHINA

Most ancient sages put forward the concept of "unity of form and Shen," such as Lao Tzu's "harmony of nutrient qi and corporeal soul," Mo Tzu's "unity of physique and knowledge," Chuang Tzu's "soma protecting psyche," Xunzi's "Shen coming after body," and Fan Zhen's "material entity of form and attributes of Shen," etc. These serve as original theory guidance on holism of life – "unity of form and Shen" in TCM psychology.

(3) "THEORY ON HEART GOVERNING" IN ANCIENT CHINA

"Theory on heart governing" is the origin of thought that "heart controlling Shen," a core theory in TCM psychology. Since Mencius proposed that "Heart plays a role in thinking," almost all the ancients considered heart as the organ for contemplation. What is the essence of theory on heart governing? *Huai Nan Zi*, a philosophical classic of Taoism, writes, "Heart is the master of body, while Shen is the most precious part." It means, the key point is not the shape of heart, but the hidden treasure-Shen. More clearly, Wang Shouren (a grandmaster of heart theory in Ming Dynasty) put forward that "Heart is not a piece of flesh, but anywhere perceptual" and "Heart is the ruler of body" (*Chuan Xi Lu*, a classic of Wang Shouren's philosophy). What is the ruler of body? Shen. To conclude, the essence of theory on heart governing is Shen. Nowadays, some scholars propose "theory on brain" and consider "theory on heart governing" unscientific. A major dispute lies in organic brain and visceral heart, but actually they are unified in the point that Shen governs life.

(4) TRADITIONAL CHINESE THINKING: IMAGE THINKING

Image thinking is fully applied to explain theory of TCM psychology. It is a traditional way of thinking for the Chinese nation and greatly influences mindset of the Oriental. Image thinking was formed early in ancient China. For instance, *I Ching* (*Book of Changes*) makes the eight diagrams of Tai-Chi and Hetu Luoshu (an atlas of galaxy) models for image of Heaven and Earth, and thus writes "to master laws of nature and to compare condition of everything." Chapter *Xici* says, "Books cannot clearly express words, not to mention thoughts," and "Creating images help convey ideas." It means, "image" can be used for clearer explanation. Embodying our ancestors' wisdom, the thinking mode made a valuable contribution to exploring the unknown and creating a high level of civilization in ancient China. Image thinking is the original thinking method in traditional Chinese medicine, such as visceral manifestation theory, meridian and collateral theory, etc. Therefore, as the psychology of traditional Chinese medicine, TCM psychology upholds image thinking, which is reflected in core concepts like "Shen (Spirit)" and "Heart."

(5) "THEORY ON EMOTION AND DESIRE" IN ANCIENT CHINA

The essence of "theory on emotion and desire" plays an important role in emotional doctrine of TCM psychology. In *Book of Rites*, "Desire and disgust occupy most of one's heart" indicates the bipolarity of emotion. Mencius once said, "Temperament originates from all things and develops into four virtues when combined with emotions." Xunzi said, "Temperament is inherent and reflected in emotions." Both sentences point out the relationship between temperament and emotion. Emotion embodies human nature since everyone has his moods. Xunzi also said, "Heart making choices is called thought," emphasizing the leading role of heart in mental activities. *On Balance* says, "Emotions of the mortal depends on gain and loss. Gain refers to happiness, while loss refers to anger." It clearly states the relationship between human's mental activities and realization of "desire." All of these discourses are vital viewpoints on emotional doctrine of TCM psychology.

(6) "THEORY ON WILL AND THOUGHT" IN ANCIENT CHINA

Most psychological ideas in *The Inner Canon of the Yellow Emperor* concern cognition and emotion, with few related to will and thought. The doctrine of will and thought in TCM psychology is mainly compiled from essence of "theories on will and thought" in ancient classics. It includes the definition, process, function and cultivation of will and thought, and relationships among will, thought, emotion, and cognition. It is particularly emphasized that the process of will and thought is dominated by Heart Shen (Spirit). Words that "will is the destination of heart" and "thought is the revelation of heart" help summarize the doctrine of will and thought in TCM psychology as "theory of heart affecting will and thought."

(7) "THEORY ON HUMAN NATURE" IN ANCIENT CHINA

In ancient China, there is no concept of personality. Its connotation belongs to category of "human nature." Therefore, essence of "theory on human nature" played an important role in the personality doctrine of TCM psychology. As is said in *The Analects of Confucius*, "By nature, men are nearly alike; by practice, they get to be wide apart." It emphasizes that although formation of personality is related to natural endowment, many acquired factors directly affect the process, and thus people's personality differs from each other. The classification of "aggressive," "conservative," and "unbiased" is the prototype of personality classification in TCM psychology, which acts according to the amount of yin and yang. In *Records of Personages* by Liu Shao (a thinker in the Three Kingdoms Period), it puts forward that "acquiring qi of yin and yang and developing personality of softness and rigidity," "acquiring yin and yang to establish one's personality while obtaining five elements to form one's shape," "everything has its own shape and shape contains spirit." These words imply the ideas of personality and physique, which are essential in the personality doctrine of TCM psychology. Hence, the doctrine is also called "theory on personality and physique."

(8) "THEORY ON DREAM" IN ANCIENT CHINA

Ancient sages had profound discussions on dream. Mo Tzu said that "dream is what one experiences when sleeping" and "without consciousness." He emphasized that dream occurs during sleep. People still have conscious activity when asleep, but instead of autonomic awareness in awakening state, it is unspontaneous consciousness. Xuncious even put it more vividly, "Heart dreams when one sleeps, rests when one relaxes, works when one ponders." He demonstrated the psychological nature of dream from the relationship between Spirit and ethereal soul. "Ethereal soul follows Spirit forward and backward." Spirit monitors activities of ethereal soul. In the daytime, ethereal soul follows Spirit outside and "works"; at night, heart sleeps and Spirit returns, letting the guard down. As a result, the out-of-control ethereal soul "rests" and explores through dream secretly. There are many kinds of dreams in ancient China, like "Six Dreams" in *Rituals of Zhou*. These ideas are of great significance to the doctrine of dream in TCM psychology.

1.4   TCM Psychology is Guided by TCM Theory

As the psychology of traditional Chinese medicine, TCM psychology is guided by TCM theory. TCM theoretical system was basically established by *The Inner Canon of the Yellow Emperor*, including holism of "correspondence between nature and human," yin-yang theory, five phase theory, visceral manifestation theory, meridian and collateral theory, cause and mechanism of disease, therapeutic principle, and methods of treatment, etc. All of basic concepts and theories in TCM psychology are explained by TCM theory.

1.4.1 TCM interpretation of basic concepts

(1) CONCEPT OF SHEN

Shen is the core concept of TCM psychology that embodies image thinking. It was constantly developed in ancient times. *Origin of Chinese Characters* explains "Shen" as "producer of everything," indicating that originally "Shen" refers to a personified god ruling the world. In the Spring and Autumn Period and the Warring States Period, with the development of productive forces, people realized that "yin and yang" is the ruler of natural changes in heaven and earth. Thus, *Book of Changes* writes, "Shen is unpredictability of yin and yang." Afterwards, people further realized regularity of yin-yang changes. Thus, concept of Shen ascends to a philosophical level, in which intrinsic laws of Nature dominates changes of everything. In *The Inner Canon of the Yellow Emperor*, Shen refers to objective laws that governs changes of heaven, earth, and human beings, taking off the mysterious cloak of God.

The Inner Canon of the Yellow Emperor divides Shen into two categories.

1) Shen of heaven and earth: Xu hao, a scholar in the Qing Dynasty, noted that "heaven and earth beget all things, and the master of things is Shen." It exactly means the objective laws governing changes of heaven and earth. *The Inner Canon of the Yellow Emperor* mentions many times that Shen of heaven and earth is yin and yang. "Yin and yang are the way of heaven and earth, great outlines of everything, parents of change, root and beginning of birth and destruction, and palace of mental activities." Although yin and yang are intangible, Nature is changing in an evident and orderly manner. It is Shen of heaven and earth who dominated the changes.

2) Shen of human body: Despite complexity, life activities of human being are methodically organized by Shen of human body. As a big world, natural changes of the universe are dominated by Shen of heaven and earth; as a small world, life activities of human beings are governed by Shen of human body. The complexity lies in various life phenomena in vitro, which occurs due to Shen of human body. Thus, Shen can be understood according to these "images." Imitating Xu Hao's words, I summarize that "human body produces many images, and the master of images is Shen." Therefore, Shen of human body refers to the symbol of life in a broad sense. *The Inner Canon of the Yellow Emperor* puts forward that "One who gains Shen is healthy while one who does not is in danger of death." Life activities include not only physiological activities featuring material and energy metabolism, but also psychological ones featuring mental consciousness, that is, Shen of human body in a narrow sense. The concept of Shen applied in TCM

psychology belongs to the narrow one-Shen at psychological level, which refers to human's mental activities.

According to levels and functions, Shen of human body is divided into five categories: spirit, ethereal soul, corporeal soul, thought, and will. According to origins, it can be distinguished as innate Shen and acquired Shen.

(2) FIVE CATEGORIES OF SHEN

1) Spirit
Spirit is the general of the five categories. "It rules ethereal soul and corporeal soul, and controls thought and will." Spirit is hidden in one's heart. In other words, "heart stores spirit." *Miraculous Pivot, Chapter Original Shen* writes, "Spirit is the fusion of yin essence and yang essence." Therefore, Spirit also symbolizes a new life reproduced by parents.

2) Ethereal Soul
Miraculous Pivot, Chapter Original Shen writes, "Ethereal soul follows Shen forward and backward." Ethereal soul is a lower-level Shen under Spirit's rule. "Forward" means future, while "backward" indicates the past. "Forward and backward" implies the past, present, and future. That is to say, corporeal soul follows Spirit to carry out consciousness activities in an awakening state. These activities include memory on the past, cognition for the present, and plan for future. However, when one sleeps, Spirit returns to heart and lets the guard down. Ethereal soul gets rid of monitoring and "rests secretly," and thus produces a special consciousness activity in an unaware state – "a trance dream with irregular changes." As Xunzi said, "Heart dreams when one sleeps, rests when one relaxes, works when one ponders." Ethereal soul is stored in liver, together with Spirit belonging to "yang Shen." Spirit is yang within yang, while ethereal soul is yin within yang.

3) Corporeal Soul
Miraculous Pivot, Chapter Original Shen writes, "Corporeal soul follows Essence outward and inward." Essence is the foundation of life. Thus, "follows Essence outward and inward" shows that corporeal soul exists with essence once a life is born, indicating the innate property. "Outward and inward" implies direction. "Outward" means from inside to outside. It refers to innate, extrovert behavior. For instance, a baby will wave, cry, and shout after birth. "Inward" means from outside to inside. It refers to instinct perception stimulated by external environment, such as pain and itch. As is said in *Classified Canon*, "Corporeal soul can be both dynamic and static,

through which pain and itch are felt." Corporeal soul is stored in lung, together with Essence belonging to yin. Thus, there is saying that "Ethereal soul is yang Shen, while corporeal soul is yin Shen."

4) Thought and Will

Miraculous Pivot, Chapter Original Shen writes, "Thought is what heart memorizes, and will is where thought is stored." This is an outward-to-inward concept of cognitive category, which refers to storage of memory. *Miraculous Pivot, Chapter Innate Viscera* writes, "Thought and will is used for ruling Spirit, gathering ethereal and corporeal soul, adapting to cold and heat, and regulate emotions." Obviously, this is an inward-to-outward concept mentioning control of ethereal and corporeal soul, mental activities, and body's adaptability to external environment. Thought and will differs from each other. *Classified Classic* writes, "Thought is what heart yearns for but still uncertain" and "Will is determined thought." Spleen stores thought and kidney stores will. Under the command of heart Spirit, thought and will are higher-level Shen regulating mental, behavioral and physiological activities, serving as strong motive forces.

(3) INNATE SHEN

1) Concept of Innate Shen

Innate (Yuan) Shen is a concept against acquired (Shi) Shen. Yuan means original, so Yuan Shen is innate Shen. Shi means cognizing and identifying, so Shi Shen is acquired Shen after birth, also known as Shen of thought or desire. In *The Inner Canon of the Yellow Emperor*, the narrow sense of Shen regarding human's mental and consciousness activities is exactly acquired Shen. Although concept of innate Shen is not clearly put forward, it has already been discussed in relevant discourses. For example, "Spirit is the fusion of yin essence and yang essence." Spirit here is innate. Innate Shen exits with the birth of human being. It is infused when fertilized egg is implanted and embryo is formed. *The Inner Canon of the Yellow Emperor* writes that "Heart accommodates Shen… Human beings exist."

The concept of innate Shen was first seen in Taoism classics, and was summarized based on practical experience. *Yin Fu Ching* first put forward concept of "not Shen," saying that "people only knows mysterious Shen, but do not understand the real mystery lies in not Shen." It means that ordinary people can only understand Shen of mental thinking and emotional activities such as contemplation and desire, but cannot notice more profound Shen of unconsciousness. This kind of Shen is a special mental state perceived by cultivators after certain periods of practice. As different from normal Shen, it is called "not Shen." It was not widely used in Taoism classics until the name is changed into "Innate Shen" in *The Secret of the Golden Flower* during the Tang Dynasty. In the Song Dynasty, understanding on innate Shen was further developed. Zhang Boduan clearly pointed out in *Tsinghua Secret Jinbao Internal Alchemy Formula*, "Shen includes innate Shen and acquired Shen. Innate Shen is brilliance since birth; acquired Shen is manifestation of qi obtained after birth." It explicitly distinguished the nature of innate Shen and acquired Shen.

From current literature, concept of "Innate Shen" was introduced into traditional Chinese medicine in the Ming Dynasty by Li Shizhen. He mentioned in *Compendium of Materia Medica, Chapter Xinyi* that "brain is the palace for innate Shen." Later, Zhang Jiebin also mentioned innate Shen in *Classified Canon*, "Shen of human body is ruled by heart... Five Shen and five minds such as ethereal soul, corporeal soul, thought and will, are all transformed by innate Shen and controlled by heart." Then it was Zhang Xichun who clearly put forward concept of innate Shen and acquired Shen in the field of traditional Chinese medicine in the late Qing Dynasty and the beginning of the Republic of China. He wrote in *Integrating Chinese and Western Medicine, Chapter Interpretation of Mentality*, "Innate Shen is natural and illusory without practical thinking; acquired Shen is mysterious but tangible with consideration."

2) How to understand Innate Shen

First, we have to admit that innate Shen exists objectively. Although generally ordinary people are unaware of it, innate Shen can be perceived and even repeated in a special state, like Taoist internal alchemy process. As long as people enter the state of "tranquility and emptiness," innate Shen will appear spontaneously. As *Pulse Inspection* writes, "Innate Shen is a kind of Shen without internal thoughts producing and external ideas invading." *Collection of Martial Arts* writes. "The heart must be clear and calm, without a single thought or awareness. In emptiness, as if seeing innate Shen permeating inside, I feel that five aggregates are all empty and four limbs all disappear. Only the true self exists." When practicing qigong (deep breathing exercises), innate Shen appears on the critical point of continuous breathing, lifelessness, carelessness, ecstasy, and trance.

Secondly, we must understand the relationship between innate Shen and acquired Shen. Both are Shen of human body, but there are differences in nature. Innate Shen is thoughtless, while acquired Shen is full of consideration; innate Shen is inborn natural spirit, while acquired Shen is mysterious but tangible spirit with external cultivation. As people grow up, acquired Shen gradually develops under the influence of family, school, and social environment. People tend to gain more knowledge and have more thoughts and desires. Thus, despite the congenital advantage, innate Shen is blocked and suppressed as acquired Shen strengthens. This is exactly what

Zhang Boduan said, "Acquired Shen is temperament nature; innate Shen is inborn property," and "origin is slight while temperament is outstanding." Therefore, innate Shen and acquired Shen is unity of opposites.

Innate Shen is kind of inborn Shen of human body. Then how to understand "innate"? Everything related to life before birth should be regarded as innate. Not only everything the biological parents endows and inherits is innate, but what the parents inherited from the grandparents should also be considered as innate. In this way, it can be traced back to ancestors, the original ancestors of mankind, and even the origin of life. All of these genes inherited from generation to generation, like the aura of eternal existence in Taixu (Taosim), should be regarded as innate. As *Book of Life* puts it, "After intersection of parents, a bit of aura… Innate Shen comes from Taixu." Innate Shen comes from parents, and even the origin of life. It can be traced back to the root of life, because the imprint exists throughout the evolution of mankind. Exploring the origin of innate Shen is a broad and profound process that requires multidisciplinary collaboration that involves genetics, anthropology, and theory of evolution at least.

For further understanding, current views on innate Shen are listed as follows:

a) In Buddhism, the first six consciousness (eyes, ears, nose, tongue, body, mind) belongs to acquired Shen. When achieving the eighth consciousness (Alaya), acquired Shen is blocked and Innate Shen appears.

b) In modern psychology, some consider innate Shen as subconscious. But we think it is inaccurate since subconscious is unrealized consciousness, still belonging to the category of consciousness. However, innate Shen is inborn "primitive unconscious" with obvious natural attributes.

c) In *Psychology of Consciousness of Returning to the Root*, written by Professor Sun Zexian, the author treats innate Shen as "consciousness of returning to the root," emphasizing the inborn natural attributes.

d) Based on theory of motivation, some put forward that innate Shen is a powerful "origin of internal driving force." Human life is controlled by it unconsciously. This is where life potential lies. It can be considered that innate Shen is the energy source of instinctive life activities, such as self-stability and adjustment ability, self-healing ability of diseased organisms, ability to avoid harm and seek benefit in emergencies, ability to comprehend action and inaction, etc.

e) Innate Shen is also understood from "genes," "genetic material," "genetic information," and "internal factors and laws of human development and changes."

f) Professor Pan Yi wrote in 2012, "Innate Shen is the most basic existence of human beings. It is the ruler of life activities, with internal mechanism and law since birth. It can be regarded as the spiritual mark that witnessed generations of mankind obtaining certain important basic attributes in the process of adapting to nature and society and evolving themselves.

3) How to develop Innate Shen

Innate Shen is of great significance to human life. It can stimulate physiological potential of human body and regulate viscera, meridians, qi and blood, achieving balance between yin and yang, and keeping the organism in optimal state.

Since innate Shen is so important to human life and physical and mental health, how to develop it? I elaborated on this issue in my paper titled "Exploitation of 'Yuan Shen' in Chinese Medical Psychology," which is published in the 9th issue of *Chinese Journal of Basic Medicine in Traditional Chinese Medicine* in 2011. According to cultivation experience of ancient Taoism and Buddhism, the basic principle of developing innate Shen is to restrain acquired Shen. With the expansion of acquired Shen, desire becomes so big that it blocks innate Shen. Therefore, developing innate Shen is to fight against it, that is, to control one's desire to liberate innate Shen. "Taking no action to approach the state. Then the driving force of human body development is innate Shen." (*Tsinghua Secret Jinbao Internal Alchemy Formula*) At this moment innate Shen appears.

Traditional methods of developing Innate Shen include Confucian moral cultivation, Taoist cultivation, and Buddhist meditation. Confucian moral cultivation is also a method for refinement of heart, in which desires are controlled to a minimum and innate Shen is liberated. Taoist cultivation and Buddhist meditation also controls acquired Shen to liberate innate Shen. Besides, practicing qigong under correct guidance can also achieve liberation. However, it is impossible for everyone to practice Taoism and meditation. And it does not accord with the actual situation of today's society. Therefore, the task of TCM psychology is to develop technical means for modern life and clinical application to liberate innate Shen and exploit potential, thereby improving people's physical and mental health.

1.4.2 Application of Yin-Yang Theory and Five Phase Theory

As TCM basic theory, yin-yang theory and five phase theory are fully used for interpretation of important theory and provide guidance on clinical application in TCM psychology.

(1) INTERPRETATION ON HOLISM OF "NATURE, SOCIETY, AND HUMAN"

Yin and yang summarize the "three powers" of heaven, earth, and man. It expanded holism of correspondence between nature and human into a "three-power holism" theory, in which man corresponds to heaven and earth, and stays harmonious with society. Therefore, the "three-power holism" theory is established in TCM psychology.

The five phase theory divides the human life system into five interacting subsystems: wood, fire, earth, metal, and water. It applies "image thinking" in ancient China and integrates heaven, earth and man into the five-element system. Instead of being enclosed in human body, the five-element system of human life is open and closely connected with the universe, nature, and society. Identical qi gathers and interconnects in the same system, while different systems engenders, restrains, overwhelms, and rebels against each other. This is the theoretical basis of "three-power holism" theory in TCM psychology, which guides clinical treatment such as emotion therapy, music therapy, color therapy, etc.

(2) INTERPRETATION ON THEORY OF "FIVE VISCERA AND EMOTION"

The Inner Canon of the Yellow Emperor writes, "In universe, there are five elements governing five positions to produce wind, cold, summerheat, dampness, dryness, and fire; In human body, there are five viscera transforming five qi to generate joy, anger, anxiety, thought, and fear." This is the theoretical basis of "five viscera and emotion" theory in TCM psychology. Using the five phase theory, it connects five viscera with five emotions. Liver is affected by anger, Heart by joy, Spleen by thought, Lung by sorrow, and Kidney by fear. These are related "emotion-viscera" theories.

(3) INTERPRETATION ON THEORY OF "YIN, YANG, AND DREAM"

The yin-yang mechanism of sleeping includes yin-yang change during day and night, yin-yang inward and outward movement of defensive qi, and yin-yang activity of Heart Shen (Spirit). The occurrence and image of dreams are also closely related to changes of yin, yang, and five elements.

(4) THEORETICAL BASIS FOR PERSONALITY CLASSIFICATION IN TCM PSYCHOLOGY

Personality classification in TCM psychology is based on yin, yang, and five elements. According to amount of yin and yang, people can be divided into "five yin-yang patterns," namely greater yang, lesser yang, balanced yin-yang, lesser yin, and greater yin. According to characteristics of five elements, people can be divided into "twenty-five yin-yang types." *The Inner Canon of the Yellow Emperor* writes, "After five elements (metal, wood, water, earth, and fire) are established, different people should be identified by five different complexions and five different body shapes. Hence there are twenty-five kinds of people."

1.4.3 Application of Visceral Manifestation Theory

Visceral manifestation theory is the most prominent embodiment of image thinking in TCM theory. What is "visceral manifestation"? Wang Bing, a doctor in the Tang Dynasty, noted that "viscera indicates hiding inside" and "manifestation means what can be seen from outside." In other words, internal "viscera" can be learnt from external "manifestation." Therefore, viscera in TCM are not organs in anatomy, but zang organs indicating images. In TCM psychology, visceral manifestation theory is mainly used in Heart."

The core theory of TCM psychology is "Heart controlling Shen." "Heart" refers to manifestation indicating images, which includes two parts in summary: Heart governing blood and vessels; Heart controlling Shen. In psychology, the main research content is manifestation of "Heart controlling Shen." *The Inner Canon of the Yellow Emperor* writes, "Heart is the organ similar to the monarch and is responsible for spirit and mental activity."

In *Miraculous Pivot, Chapter Pathogen*, it points out connotation of "Heart controlling Shen," "Heart is the master of five viscera and six bowels, and the house of spirit." It means Heart is the ruler of human physical and psychological activities. Thus, "Heart controlling Shen" means Heart dominates whole life activities. Mental and physical activities are under the dominance of "Heart Shen," which is the theoretical basis for monism of "mind-body correlation" in TCM psychology. Specifically, the connotation includes the following aspects.

1) Heart is the master of five viscera and six bowels, ruling coordination in functions of these organs. *The Inner Canon of the Yellow Emperor* writes, "If the master is in calm and peace, twelve officials will work well; otherwise, they will be in disorder."
2) Heart leads cognition of the objective world. *The Inner Canon of the Yellow Emperor* writes, "Heart lets things grow and change naturally" and "Heart exists when things are under examination."
3) Heart dominates emotional activities. In *Confucians' Duties to Parents*, it says "five emotions are all produced by Heart." *Classified Classic* also writes, "All emotions are controlled by Heart."

4) Heart guides will and thought, that is, "will is the destination of Heart" and "thought is the revelation of Heart."

1.5 Basic Theoretical Framework of TCM Psychology

As the theoretical support for construction of a new discipline, basic theory of TCM psychology is quite important. Its research content includes guiding ideology, core theories, TCM interpretation of psychological phenomena, etc. Constructing the basic theoretical framework of TCM psychology should cover all of the above. Construction of framework contributes to continuous enrichment, development and improvement on basic theory of TCM psychology. It clarifies that guiding ideology of TCM psychology is theory on unity of form and Shen and three-power holism. The core theory is theory on Heart controlling Shen. Interpretation of psychological process is theory on Heart Shen cognition and perception, five viscera and emotion, and Heart affecting will and thought. Besides, there are theory on "yin, yang, and dream" demonstrating dream psychology and theory on personality and constitution elaborating personal characteristics.

1.5.1 Theory on Unity of Form and Shen

Holism is the guiding ideology of TCM psychology. Theory on unity of form and Shen expounds holism in nature of life. Through explaining relationship between form and Shen, it emphasizes materiality of spiritual activities and the leading role of Shen in life activities. Thus, the theory is the basis for fundamental theory of TCM psychology.

(1) CONCEPT OF FORM AND SHEN

"Form" here not only refers to macroscopic body shape, but more importantly, microcosmic essence and qi. "Shen" here is spirit of human body, emphasizing the "master" of life. "Shen" is a concept of image thinking and includes root and branch. The root of Shen is dominance of life, while the branch of Shen is phenomenon of life. This is the concept I summarize as "human body produces many images, and the master of images is Shen."

(2) Relationship between Form and Shen

The relationship between form and spirit is that Shen originates from and relies on form (essence) to exist; meanwhile, Shen is the master of form, controlling body and qi to dominate life activities. As Zhang Jiebin, a famous doctor in the Ming Dynasty, said, "Form is the carrier of Shen, and Shen is the function of form. Form cannot live without Shen, and Shen cannot exist without form." (*Classified Classic*) Therefore, the feature of life is that "body and Shen are combined in harmony," which is emphasized in *The Inner Canon of the Yellow Emperor*. On the contrary, death is that "Shen and qi have gone, leaving body shape alone."

(3) Clinical Significance of Theory on Unity of Form and Shen

Theory on unity of form and Shen is quite essential to clinical diagnosis, treatment and life nurturing in TCM. As the master of life, Shen is paid more attention in four examinations (inspection, listening and smelling, inquiry, and palpation) of TCM. Clinical treatment also emphasizes the leading role of Shen in life activities. Therefore, *The Inner Canon of the Yellow Emperor* writes that "normal doctors treat form while skilled ones regulate Shen," putting treatment of Shen in the first place. As is said in Plain Questions, Chapter Protecting the Body, "The first thing is to treat Shen, second to preserve health, and third to learn flavors and nature of medicinals..." Since life is unity of form and Shen, life nurturing should start from two aspects: one is to cultivate Shen, and the other is to regulate body shape. As Shen is the master of form, cultivating Shen should be the first priority.

1.5.2 *Three-power Holism Theory*

Three-power holism theory is to put the unity of human body and Shen into the external environment, and thus to explore the relationship among life activities (including physical and psychological activities), nature and changes of society. It emphasizes holism of correspondence between human and nature, and harmony between human and society.

Named as "three-power holism theory," it applies doctrine of "three powers" from *Book of Changes* for interpretation. Three powers refer to heaven, earth, and man. In *Book of Changes*, each hexagram has upper, middle, and lower lines as representative symbols. Upper line means heaven, lower line means earth, and lines of man lies in the middle of heaven and earth. This shows a universe model of correspondence between human and nature. However, the model is an imperfect, static one as it fails to reflect change of yin and yang.

"Yin and yang are the way of heaven and earth and great outlines of everything." After added change of yin and yang, the original model become a new one with six lines, forming a dynamic model of 64 hexagrams that can reflect yin-yang movements of three powers (heaven, earth and man). The model is called "Way of three powers." As is said in *Interpretation of Changes, Chapter Explaining Hexagrams*, "Way of heaven is yin and yang; way of earth is softness and rigidity; way of human is benevolence and righteousness. With three powers and yin and yang combined, six lines in *Book of Change* become a hexagram." Obviously, man in three powers no longer refers to an individual person, but a society composed of groups with different human natures. Therefore, what way of three powers integrates is holism of man, nature and social environment. Now let's talk about the psychological effects of yin-yang change in heaven, earth and man.

(1) Yin-yang Change in Heaven and Psychology

Yin-yang change in heaven mainly refer to changes of day and night, waxing and waning, seasons and years, and five circuits and six qi, which are caused by movements of the sun, moon, and stars. By influencing changes of yin, yang, qi, and blood in human body, these changes affect human's psychological activities.

Yin-yang change of day and night affects biological clock of sleeping and ups and downs of one's mood. Yin-yang change of waxing and waning have a more notable impact on emotions. When the moon is full, human body's blood and qi are most vigorous, which means people tend to lose control of their emotions and have deviant behavior. Therefore, in some countries the night of full moon is called "Devil's Night." Spring and summer refer to yang, while autumn and winter refer to yin. Yin-yang change of four seasons can affect blood and qi in human body, and thus mental activities. As is said in *The Inner Canon of the Yellow Emperor*, "One should conform with four seasons to regulate Shen." Five circuits and six qi are yin-yang change of a sixty-year circle. In *The Inner Canon of the Yellow Emperor*, it records different syndromes of abnormal emotions in symptoms of different sexagenary cycles. Natural disaster caused by abnormal weather changes is an important cause of psychological trauma. Abnormal astronomical change affects animals' behavior, and so is human psychology. Therefore, it is suggested not to determine important matters due to disturbance in cognitive ability.

(2) Yin-yang Change in Earth and Psychology

As is mentioned in *Book of Changes*, yin-yang change in earth mainly lies in softness and rigidity of water and soil, which are related to many factors such as territorial positions, topography, and geographical environment. "The unique features of a local environment always give special characteristics to its inhabitants." Hence, one's constitution and temperament will be different because of water and soil with different attributes.

In *Plain Questions, Chapter Different Situations and Suitable solutions*, it talks about five different directions: east, south, center, west, and north. Due to different degrees in softness and wetness of soil and water, people have different constitutions They have distinct symptoms and thus different treatments are applied. Although temperament is not mentioned here, it must differ in various regions according to theory on "unity of form and Shen." "Terrain of the northwest is high while the southeast is low." The northwest is a dry place, where people are bold and straightforward; the southeast is a soft place, where people tend to be delicate and gentle in words and deeds.

The difference is also reflected in culture. For instance, Kun Opera and Yue Opera produce completely different feelings from those of Shaanxi Opera and Bangzi Opera. *Loess Plateau* in the northwest and *From Heaven Fallen an Angel Sister Lin* in the southeast, two tunes of entirely different styles, reflect influence of "softness and rigidity of earth" on psychology in temperament.

(3) Yin-yang Change in Man and Psychology

"Way of man" is a broad concept that has different meanings in different categories. In Buddhism, way of human refers to one of the three good ways of reincarnation in the six realms (nature, man, asura, animal, beast, and hell); in ethics, it refers to principle of behavior or social norm; in humanities, it refers to humanism, that is, to care for lives and to respect personality and human rights, In ancient China, way of intersecting between male and female, yin and yang, is also called way of man.

Way of man, mentioned in *Book of Changes*, is a concept corresponding to heaven and earth, which is also way of yin and yang. *The Inner Canon of the Yellow Emperor* writes, "Those who master Way know astronomy from heaven, geography from earth, and principles of interpersonal relationship from man." Although Way is intangible, knowing astronomy can help understand way of heaven; knowing geography can help learn way of earth; knowing principles of interpersonal relationship can help grasp way of man. Therefore, way of man here refers to human affairs, that is, all matters in human society. *Book of Changes* says, "Way of human is benevolence and righteousness." It reflects Confucianism in three-power theory, using the contradiction and unity between "benevolence" and "righteousness" to explain yin-yang change in way of man.

Yin-yang changes in man are embodied in social and interpersonal factors ranging from social reforms, wars and chaos, to personal life events and fickleness of human relationships. These are originally the most important psychological stress, which can affect human psychology. Undesirable emotions include great joy, great sorrow, fear, thought, worry, depression, anger, etc. These will seriously affect physical and mental health, and thus harmony between people and society.

In addition, different social environments also affect human psychology. Educational environment, including family education, school education, and social atmosphere, all affect acquired temperament and personality shaping; music also exerts influence. In *Book of Rites, Chapter Music*, it expounds music regulating psychology. By influencing one's will and thought, music can destroy a country or rejuvenate a nation. Great Wind Song by Liu Bang, the emperor of the Han Dynasty, enhances morale and helps establish the Han world. *The Internationale* promotes world communist movement. *March of the Volunteers* not only inspired the fighting spirit of whole nation during the anti-Japanese period, but because of its exciting melody, it still encourages us today to strive for realizing the Chinese dream of national rejuvenation.

Colors can make people have different psychological feelings. It is reported that once a black bridge was built in London, England. As black is a negative color making people melancholic and fearful, suicides on this bridge had occurred from time to time since construction. Later, the problem was discovered, so the color was changed into blue, and thus number of suicide cases around the bridge decreased significantly. Therefore, patients with depression should avoid staying in claustrophobic rooms. They can go out to enjoy vast sea, blue sky, green lawns and forests. Such an environment and color can help people relax and relieve depression. The influence of music and color on psychology has become theoretical basis of music therapy and color therapy in TCM psychotherapy. It also helps develop musical and environmental ways of health preservation in TCM psychology.

1.5.3 Theory on Heart Controlling Shen

Theory on heart controlling Shen is a monism doctrine using visceral image of heart to explain regulation and integration of complicated life activities in human body, which emphasizes the leading role of heart Shen in mental activities and mechanism of interaction between mind and body from a psychological perspective. It is the core theory of TCM psychology.

(1) CONCEPT OF HEART

As is mentioned before, Heart here is not merely an organ of flesh and blood, but heart with images. The concept has a profound background of traditional Chinese culture and incorporates more ideas of philosophy and psychology, and thus reflects deeper psychological meanings. In traditional Chinese culture, not only traditional Chinese medicine, but also Confucianism, Buddhism, and Taoism also divide Heart into category of spirit.

(2) Essence of Heart Controlling Shen

Essence of Heart controlling Shen is that, under the guidance of theory on unity of form and Shen, Heart of images carries Shen of human body to help it function as "master of life." Heart houses Shen and serves as the form that Shen depends on. In return, Shen functions for Heart. They reflect the relationship that "form provides material entity while Shen produces attributes and functions," which is the same as the relationship between blade and edge. As is described by Fan Zhen in *On Extinction of Shen*, "Blade and edge cannot exist without each other." Usage of Heart is exactly function of Shen residing in Heart, Heart Shen for short or only "Heart" instead.

(3) Connotation of Heart Controlling Shen

The connotation includes two major aspects, that is, "Heart is the master of five viscera and six bowels, and the house of spirit." It can be summarized as follows.

1) Heart Shen leads and regulates function of viscera. *The Inner Canon of the Yellow Emperor* writes, "Heart is the organ similar to the monarch and is responsible for spirit and mental activity... If the master is in calm and peace, twelve officials will work well; otherwise, they will be in disorder."
2) Heart Shen dominates cognitive process of the objective world. "Heart lets things grow and change naturally." This is theory on "Heart Shen cognition" and "Heart Shen perception" that will be explained later.
3) Heart Shen rules attitudes and experiences towards the objective world. The external manifestation of internal experiences is emotion. Thus, Heart Shen also regulates emotional process. As is said in *Classified Classic*, "All emotions are controlled by Heart."
4) Heart Shen guides behavior of will and thought. Will and thought originate from motivation, that is, the intention in one's heart. Behavior governed by will and thought is controlled by Heart Shen, including random movements and verbal behavior. Therefore, "Heart affecting will and thought."

5) Heart Shen commands all kinds of Shen. It is the supreme commander of all kinds of Shen. Ethereal soul, corporeal soul, will, and thought produce spiritual activities methodically under leadership of Heart Shen. As is written in *Principle and Prohibition for Medical Profession* by Yu Chang, "Heart... rules ethereal soul and corporeal soul, and controls thought and will."

(4) CLINICAL SIGNIFICANCE OF HEART CONTROLLING SHEN

After decades of clinical practice, I have deeply realized that Heart Controlling Shen is important to clinical treatments. Under the guidance of this theory, I have formed my own clinical philosophy: When curing diseases, curing patient first; when curing patient, cure his Heart first.

1) Cure patient first: We should realize that diseases occur on people, so people should be the subject. In clinical diagnosis and treatment, we should not focus on pathogen. Instead, people should be the priority. Improving human body's self-regulation ability and resistance to diseases should be paid more attention.
2) Cure patient's Heart first: Man is an organic unity of form and Shen. As the master of form, Shen dominates life activities and governs human body's self-regulation ability and resistance to diseases. Hence, treating Shen is essential. Shen resides in Heart and Heart houses Shen, so treat Shen is to treat Heart.

1.5.4 Theory on Heart Shen Cognition

Theory on Heart Shen cognition is a cognitive theory in TCM psychology.

(1) CONCEPT OF COGNITION

Cognition is a process in which people learn objective things. In philosophical category, cognitive theory is also called "epistemology." Cognition was called "knowledge and contemplation" in ancient China, or "knowing" for short. It can be divided into two types: one is "knowledge of seeing and hearing," that is, the primary stage of people's cognitive process – perceptual experience. The other is "knowledge of virtue and nature," the advanced stage of rational experience. Knowledge of seeing and hearing can be divided into "real knowledge" and "common knowledge." Real knowledge refers to one's personal and direct experience, while common knowledge refers to indirect experience obtained through learning.

The advanced stage of cognition is also called "contemplation." "Contemplation" means to ponder over what has been perceived, and to form a concept. Ancient Chinese thinkers had a deep understanding of "contemplation" and divided it into two phases: "consideration" and "contemplation." Consideration is cogitation, which means to think over something repeatedly. "Deep consideration is contemplation." "Long contemplation leads to smart ideas." However, "smart ideas" cannot be regarded as "wisdom" yet. Only when the idea is verified through practice can it be regarded as wisdom. "Wisdom is to deal with things based on contemplation."

(2) EMERGENCE OF COGNITION

Cognizing objective things requires two factors: subject and object.

Subject refers to the normal cognitive organs that a person must have, including sensory organs and thinking organ. Eyes, tongue, ears, nose, and body are sensory organs. Thinking organ is mostly considered as brain, but traditional Chinese culture takes heart. As Mencius said, "Heart is the official of thinking."

Object refers to external things existing objectively. It is the source of cognition. Cognitive process cannot be carried out without object, which is the fundamental difference between epistemology of materialism and idealism. In addition, another prerequisite of cognition is that subject and object must interact with each other, which is so called "acceptance" and "regulation." Objects must be existent and accessible. Hence, Xunzi put forward that "essence and qi interact with external things" and "external things are perceived and responded by heart."

(3) PROCESS OF COGNITION

Miraculous Pivot, Chapter Original Shen, expounds human's cognition process, "Heart regulates things. Thought is what heart memorizes, and will is where thought is stored. Consideration is to accumulate thoughts and make change. Contemplation is to expand consideration. Wisdom is to deal with matters based on contemplation." From "regulating things" to "dealing with matters," the cognitive process emphasizes that material comes the first, and that cognition needs to be tested in practice, which is epistemology of materialism. The discourse divides cognitive process into six levels, from low to high: regulating things, will, thought, consideration, contemplation, and wisdom. It demonstrates whole process of cognition: perception → impression → experience accumulation → concept formation → creative thinking → theory-guided practice. It emphasizes that Heart is the place for things growing, and the process of cognition is under dominance of Heart Shen from beginning to end. Therefore, Heart is defined as the center of cognition. Now let's analyze the process.

1) "Heart regulates things." Heart is responsible for perceiving external objects from the very beginning of cognition. It receives external information through eyes, ears, nose, tongue, and body. The information received by five sensory organs must be transmitted to Heart for further perception.

2) "Thought is what heart memorizes." After transmission, Heart records information and forms reflection of the external object. When senses separate from object, reflection still exists in Heart, which is so-called impression. But at that time impression does not reflect essence of things, so it is named as superficial image. In TCM, it can also be called image of Heart, or image of thinking.

3) "Will is where thought is stored." On the basis of "thinking," images formed by perception are stored from time to time. More accumulations mean a stage of experience gathering in the course of perception.

4) "Consideration is to accumulate thoughts and make change." Consideration is an important period in which perceptual knowledge develops into rational one. "The extreme of things is called change." On the basis of "will," Heart Shen can fully process accumulated materials through analysis, synthesis, abstraction, and generalization, forming concepts that reflect essence of things. This is known as process of consideration. At this moment, cognition has undergone a qualitative change and digs deep into essence.

5) "Contemplation is to expand consideration." "Expand" means to ponder over issues repeatedly and to plan for the future based on consideration. It is a creative process in which Heart Shen uses formed concepts to judge and reason about the future.

6) "Wisdom is to deal with things based on contemplation." The phase of contemplation is still at theoretical level. Whether cognition is correct and conforms to reality still needs to be tested in practice. "Practice is the criterion of truth." Cognition can be considered correct only if things are successfully handled under the guidance of this principle. And this is true wisdom.

These are discourses of cognition in *The Inner Canon of the Yellow Emperor*. It should be emphasized that the entire process of cognition is governed by Heart. In perception stage, one must carefully observe external objects. In thinking stage, one must attentively keep images in mind. In consideration and contemplation stage, one must prudently think and analyze ideas. Therefrom, one can have knowledge and confidence in his Heart.

1.5.5 *Theory on Heart Shen Perception*

On the basis of theory on Heart Shen cognition, theory on Heart Shen perception focuses on the sensory process of Heart and emphasizes the leading role of Heart Shen in perceptual activities. Human's perceptual experience is the primary stage of cognition. It is a process in which Heart receives external information perceived by sensory organs and produces corresponding reaction. In process of perception, sensory organs only serve as information receptors, and the leader is Heart Shen.

(1) PERCEPTION OF FIVE SENSES

Eyes are receptors of visual information. The relationship between eyes and viscera is that "Liver opens into the eyes." However, visual information received by eyes must be transmitted to Heart to form corresponding visual perception. Therefore, *Standards for Syndrome Identification and Treatment* writes, "The eyes are opened by Liver but used by Heart."

Ears are receptors of auditory information. The relationship between ears and viscera is that "Kidney opens into the ears." However, auditory information received by ears must be transmitted to Heart to form corresponding auditory perception. Therefore, *Prescriptions for Rescuing Lives* writes, "Kidney qi is connected with ears, and Heart indirectly opens into ears."

Nose is receptor of olfactory information. The Lung opens into the nose. However, olfactory information received by nose must be transmitted to Heart to form corresponding olfactory perception. Therefore, *Effective Formulas* by Li Dongyuan writes, "Nose is the orifice of Lung and function of Heart."

Tongue is receptor of gustatory information. The Heart opens into the tongue. However, sense of taste still have to be produced through gustatory information received by tongue transmitting to Heart.

(2) PERCEPTION OF BODY

Due to depth and features, there are different receptors regarding somatosensory, which can be collectively named as "body." Sense of pain is the most representative somatosensory, which can be classified as superficial or deep.

Superficial pain is a kind of skin sensation, whose receptors are located in skin. After reaching the skin, external painful stimuli will be transmitted to Heart to perceive pain, known as "pain originating from Heart."

Stimuli of deep pain comes from inner body. Mechanism of pain formation is more complicated, but still closely related to Heart Shen. *The Inner Canon of the*

Yellow Emperor says, "Most pains, itches, and sores come from Heart." Wang Bing, a doctor in the Tang Dynasty, further noted, "Calmness of Heart results in slight pain, while restlessness aggravates it." Therefore, level of pain tolerance is closely related to state of Heart Shen. Legend has it that during the Three Kingdoms period, Guan Gong "scraped bones to clear poison." As a great hero with a tenacious will, he faced it calmly without fear, showing high level of pain tolerance. Regulating state of Heart Shen is of great significance to improving clinical efficacy of pain treatment.

(3) Perception of Acupuncture

Needling sensation in acupuncture is a special kind of perception. It is also called "arrival of qi." "The main point of acupuncture is to obtain qi and to take effect." Thus, needling sensation is the key to curative effect of acupuncture. Whether qi arrives is closely related to Heart Shen. "Qi moves when Shen works." Active state of Shen can result in smooth movement of qi, and thus faster and stronger needling sensation. Otherwise, it will be difficult obtain qi. Vitality of Shen is closely connected with personality and physique. In clinical practice, regulating Shen is quite important, which is shown in *The Inner Canon of the Yellow Emperor* that "Treating Shen is the first priority in acupuncture."

(4) Abnormal Perception

As "Heart controls Shen," the key to whether perception can correctly reflect objective things lies in whether perception of Heart Shen is normal. When Heart Shen works well, perception can be produced correctly. If Heart Shen has problem in perception, it will engender wrong sensation. Delusion is wrong perception that "comes from existing objects," which is related to distance, position, light, physical and biological factors, and especially psychological factors. Illusion is wrong perception that "comes from nothing," which is closely related to Heart Shen. Recurring illusions are manifestations of disorders in Heart Shen, which should be paid serious attention in diagnosis and treatment of mental illness.

1.5.6 Theory on Five Viscera and Emotion

This is emotional theory of TCM psychology. Emotion is a collective term for Seven Emotions and Five Minds, and generalization of sentiment and emotion in TCM. Theory on five viscera and emotion applies TCM theory to explain sentimental process of human being, correlation between emotion and internal organs, and how emotional factors cause and cure diseases. The theory is so named as it highlights relationship between emotion and viscera, embodying characteristics of emotional theory in TCM psychology.

(1) Correlation between Emotion and Internal Organs

Let's explain the relationship between emotion and viscera from the following aspects.

1) Emotion is produced through qi transformation of five viscera

The Inner Canon of the Yellow Emperor clearly put forward that "In human body, there are five viscera transforming five qi to generate joy, anger, anxiety, thought, and fear." In other words, emotion is a sentimental process based on qi transformation of five viscera. Everyone has his own emotion, and emotional activities are common in human life. When one is emotionally stimulated, qi movement of viscera is activated and produces corresponding emotional changes, which are manifested through various expressions and acts. Emotional stimulus mainly refers to inner experience of whether people's desires and needs are satisfied. As "Heart is great master of five viscera and six bowels," the experience will act on five viscera separately and affect activities of qi transformation, which is reflected through corresponding changes in expressions and behavior.

2) Correspondence between emotion and five viscera

"Five viscera transform five qi to generate joy, anger, anxiety, thought, and fear." Emotions are produced and shown outside when internal organs first work inside. Five viscera have a corresponding relationship with five emotions, that is, Liver to anger, Heart to joy, Spleen to thought, Lung to sorrow (anxiety), and Kidney to fear. This is because Heart acts on the corresponding viscera according to different types of emotional stimulation, resulting in different qi movements.

3) Excessive emotion does harm to five viscera

"Excessive" here has two meanings. One means too strong, that is, emotional change is too intense. The other means too long, that is, although change is not intense, it lasts for too long. Both excessive intensity and duration of emotional change can harm five viscera and cause illness, which is the so-called seven-emotion causes in theory on TCM etiology. There is a regular pattern in seven emotions causing diseases. Since emotions are transformed by qi of five viscera, they first inhibit qi transformation, leading to disorder in qi movements, and thus injury of five viscera.

Generally, emotions do harm to corresponding viscera, that is, anger to Liver, joy to Heart, thought to Spleen, sorrow to Lung, and fear to Kidney. Furthermore, as Heart controls Shen, all emotions are first produced through inner experiences. Therefore, excessive emotions can all damage Heart. Besides, as Liver ensures the smooth flow of qi and regulates qi movement, excessive emotions will first damage qi of Liver. Hence, regardless of general law of correspondence between seven emotions and five viscera, Heart and Liver are most vulnerable to damage.

4) Mechanism for curing disease based on preponderance among emotions
Preponderance among emotions is a traditional emotional therapy in TCM psychology. It works under guidance of "theory on five viscera and emotion." Emotion of five viscera is included in five-element system. Anger belongs to Liver and wood; joy belongs to Heart and fire; thinking belongs to Spleen and earth; sorrow belongs to Lung and metal; fear belongs to Kidney and water.

Therapy of preponderance among emotions can be summarized as follows based on the law of five elements restraining each other: Anger does harm to Liver as sorrow predominates over anger; joy does harm to Heart as fear predominates over joy; thinking does harm to Spleen as anger predominates over thought; sorrow does harm to Lung as joy predominates over sorrow; fear does harm to Kidney as thought predominates over fear. The emotional treatment is verified in many ancient medicine classics and is popular among people, like the legend of "Fan Jin Passing Civil Exam."

(2) EMOTION IS GUIDED BY HEART SHEN

1) Nature of emotional activities
Nature of emotional activities a manifestation of coordinated visceral activities guided by Heart Shen. More specifically, external emotional stimuli are transmitted to Heart through five senses. Different internal experiences in Heart results in corresponding qi transformation of a certain viscus, which is manifested as emotion from the outside. In the whole process, Heart is always in a dominant position. As *Principle and Prohibition for Medical Profession* says, "Lung responds to sorrow in Heart, Spleen to thought, Liver to anger, and Kidney to fear. Five emotions are exclusively dominated by Heart."

2) State of Heart Shen affects emotional change
Besides quality and quantity of emotional stimuli, emotional change mainly depends on the state of Heart Shen, which varies in individuals and pathological

changes. State of Heart Shen is closely related to personalities and temperaments. Some are open-minded and unconstrained, and thus quickly feel relieved in face of bad emotional stimulation. However, some are narrow-minded, and shows obvious emotional changes towards trivial stimulation. When people get sick, their temperament tends to change due to change in state of Heart Shen. For example, a person with a mild temperament may become irritable after getting ill. Anger is emotion of Liver, so irritation is mostly caused by Liver qi depression or excess Liver fire. This is because ability of Heart Shen to regulate emotions is affected by diseases. Emotional differentiation can be performed based on abnormal change in emotions.

1.5.7 Theory of Heart Affecting Will and Thought

Theory of Heart affecting will and thought is taken from "will is the destination of heart" and "thought is the revelation of heart," emphasizing that human's will and thought is a psychological process dominated by Heart.

(1) CONCEPT OF WILL AND THOUGHT

Will is a term in modern psychology and one of the main contents in human psychological process. According to the connotation, will and thought were called "thought and will" (in a reverse order) in ancient China, or collectively named as "will" or "thought." There are two different conceptual categories in *The Inner Canon of the Yellow Emperor.*

Miraculous Pivot, Chapter Original Shen writes, "Thought is what heart memorizes, and will is where thought stores." It refers to an outward-to-inward psychological process. *Miraculous Pivot, Chapter Innate Viscera* writes, "Thought and will is used for ruling Spirit, gathering ethereal and corporeal soul, adapting to cold and heat, and regulate emotions." It refers to an inward-to-outward psychological process. These are two completely different concepts regarding directivity of psychological process. The former belongs to category of cognition, while the latter belongs to category of volition. Here we prefer the latter and subdivide the concept into "thought" and "will."

Classified Canon, Category of Viscera Manifestation writes, "Thought is what heart yearns for but still uncertain" and "Will is determined thought." That is to say, thought refers to undetermined intention that one has in his heart; will refers to unchangeable ambition. In the process, will is established on the basis of thought.

(2) PROCESS OF WILL AND THOUGHT

There are detailed discussions and valuable expositions on process of will and thought in ancient classics. In *History of Chinese Psychology*, Sir Gao Jue fu (a famous psychologist) summarized Confucius's syllogism on process of will and thought: "aspiration," "belief" and "perseverance." He thinks these are more comprehensive than "motivation" and "execution" in modern psychology. When sorting out doctrine of will and thought in TCM psychology, we propose that process of will and thought is guided by Heart Shen. It goes from "thought" to "thought" to "will," and to "action," and finally to "impact (gong)." Impact tests result of action on will and thought and derives from Mo Tzu's "doctrine of will and impact." Regarding evaluation system of action on will and thought, Mo Tzu puts forward the brilliant proposition that "combining aspiration and efficacy." He believes that motivation and effect should be combined to evaluate process of will and thought. As the entire process is dominated by Heart, the role of Heart at each stage can be summarized as "desire," "determination," "confidence" and "persistence." Desire is the initial stage, in which one may have multiple undetermined intentions, which is exactly "thought." Determination is that one makes up his mind to choose one target after contemplation. This is exactly setting one's aspiration based on thought. From desire to determination, it is process of thought developing into will. Confidence refers to the first psychological quality that one must possess in the execution stage after determination. It is an important manifestation of will and thought, and the first condition for smooth execution. Persistence refers to tenacity to overcome difficulties persevere to the end. It is an essential guarantee for career success and another important manifestation of will and thought.

(3) FUNCTION OF WILL AND THOUGHT

Will and thought are powerful driving forces. Their function can be summarized as follows.

1) Will and thought work as motivation for overcoming difficulties. They help produce courage to sacrifice and to solve all problems. In Mo Tzu, it says "will is foundation for courage." A strong will can generate courage to conquer everything.

2) Will and thought can control human behavior. As people's desire gradually expand with growth, Confucius proposed ethics to avoid unlimited desires and to restrict human behavior. Restricting one's behavior relies on will and thought. As Zeng Zi said, "Do not look at what is contrary to propriety; do not listen to what is contrary to propriety; do not speak what is contrary to propriety; do not

make movement which is contrary to propriety." As long as one has strong will and thought, he can manage to do so. Xunzi believed behavior can be controlled by will and thought. "Restriction, motivation, refusal, acceptance, action, and halt are all done by oneself." Without control of will and thought, people will do whatever they want, resulting in a chaotic society. Therefore, will and thought is quite essential. It greatly helps distinguish human from animals: people can use will and thought to make their behavior conform to ethics.

3) Will and thought can regulate human body. Heart Shen dominates people's spiritual activities. Being the general of "five Shen," Heart Shen "rules ethereal soul and corporeal soul, and controls thought and will." Meanwhile, *Miraculous Pivot, Chapter Innate Viscera* writes, "Thought and will is used for ruling Spirit, gathering ethereal and corporeal soul, adapting to cold and heat, and regulate emotions." Thus, Heart Shen only gives orders in dominating Spirit, ethereal soul, corporeal soul, and emotion. The executors are will and thought. They can rule Spirit, gather ethereal and corporeal soul, and regulate emotions, which are the spiritual aspect of regulating life activities. Adapting to cold and heat illustrates the physical aspect of will and thought regulating human body. Under control of tenacious will and thought, physiological limit of human being can be broken. For example, Qiu Shaoyun, a martyr during the War to Resist U.S. Aggression and Aid Korea, was able to endure pain of burning his body that ordinary people could not bear and lurked motionless in front of enemy. It is because of his tenacious will and thought for the sake of victory and safety of comrades that supported him to sacrifice himself without fear.

4) Will and thought play important roles in disease treatment and recovery. Will and thought are active consciousness, and subjective initiative of human is the most prominent embodiment. If subjective initiative is mobilized, will and thought can well "rule Spirit" and regulate human body, which is conducive to disease treatment and recovery. Otherwise, "Spirit cannot enter, will and thought cannot be stabilized, and disease cannot be cured." (*Plain Questions, Chapter Decoction*) Therefore, in clinical practice, doctors should not only use "acupuncture and medicine" to treat patients, but also fully understand function of will and thought. Active psychological counseling should be provided to improve patients' psychological quality and enhance their willpower to overcome diseases. I have elaborated on this issue in more detail in an article named "Will and Thought Functioning as a Driving Force in Clinical Treatment Should be Paid More Attention to."

1.5.8 Theory of Yin, Yang, and Dream

Theory of yin, yang, and dream in TCM psychology applies yin-yang theory in TCM to explain mechanism of sleep and dream. As one third of a person's life is spent in sleep, discussing psychological problems of sleep and dream can improve understanding of all psychological problems in life activities.

(1) SLEEP

Modern psychology believes that sleep is not only a simple end of awakening, but an active inhibition process produced by brain. Sleep is not a complete loss of awareness, but a state of consciousness opposite to being awake. Sleep is an important guarantee for physical and mental health as it helps restore energy and relieve fatigue. TCM divides sleep and awakening into yin and yang. Sleep belongs to yin, which is called "mei (寐)"; awakening belongs to yang, which is called "wu (寤)." Mei and wu are two different movements and states of yin and yang. The alternating cycle of mei and wu is the most important and outstanding pattern in life activities. It balances people's work and rest, and maintains normal life activities.

1) Yin-yang mechanism for formation of wu and mei
   a) Yin-yang change during day and night is the most basic mechanism for formation of wu and mei. "Man works at sunrise and rests at sunset." Day belongs to yang and night belongs to yin. People responds to rise and fall of yin and yang during day and night. "When yang qi fades and yin qi flourishes after nightfall, people sleep; when yin qi fades and yang qi flourishes at dawn, people get wide awake." *(Miraculous Pivot, Chapter Words of Mouth)*
   b) The second is inward and outward movement of defensive qi. In the morning, defensive qi moves from inside (yin) to outside (yang) and works in yang aspect during the day. Shen follows it to meet external things and thus gets awake. At night, defensive qi moves from outside (yang) to inside (yin) and Shen returns to inner home to rest. *Miraculous Pivot, Chapter Confusion* writes, "Defensive qi runs in yang aspect during the day and stays in yin aspect at night. People sleeps when yang qi wanes and awakes when yin qi fades." In brief, mei occurs when defensive qi flows from yang to yin, while wu occurs when it flows from yin to yang.
   c) The third is yin-yang activity of Heart Shen. Mei and wu are two different manifestations of consciousness and are dominated by Heart Shen. They are closely related to yin-yang activity of Heart Shen: Static Shen leads to mei and dynamic Shen leads to wu. As is said in *Complete Works of Jingyue*, "Mei

belongs to yin and is ruled by Shen. When Shen is stable, people sleep; when Shen is excited, people cannot rest." In brief, mei occurs when Heart Shen is in a calm yin state. Wu occurs when Heart Shen is in a restless yang state.

2) Key to maintain normal sleep

According to yin-yang mechanism for formation of wu and mei, working and resting properly in line with change of yin and yang during the day and night is the first priority to maintain a normal sleep-awaking pattern. Besides, unblocking yin-yang channels is also necessary for smooth flow of defensive qi. More importantly, yin and yang of viscera and bowels should be coordinated and upward and downward movements of qi should be balanced to make Heart Shen work well. Therefore, yin-yang coordination is the key to maintaining normal sleep. Yin-yang imbalance is the primary cause of sleep disorders and coordinating yin and yang is the main treatment.

(2) DREAM

Dream is a special psychological phenomenon that accompanies sleep.

1) Essential characteristics of dream

One of the important characteristics of dream is that dream occurs during sleep. *Mo Tzu* says, "dream is what one experiences when sleeping." *Xunzi* says, "Heart dreams when one sleeps." Both discourses pointed out that sleep is a prerequisite for dream. Thus, *Origin of Chinese Characters* explains "dream" as "sleeping with consciousness."

Dream is a special mental activity during sleep. Different from awareness activities in awakening state that takes concept as the basic element, it takes "image" as the fundamental factor. *Xunzi, Chapter Overcoming Blindness*, says "Heart dreams when one sleeps, rests when one relaxes, works when one ponders," It explains that dream cannot work on its own, but can get rid of self-control and "rests when one relaxes" spontaneously. This is different from Heart Shen planning and guiding conscious activities in awakening state.

2) Yin, yang, and occurrence of dream

Occurrence of dream is closely related to yin-yang changes in human body.

a) Dream and yin-yang sleep depth

As dream accompanies sleep, periodic changes in depth of sleep directly affect occurrence of dream. Sleep belongs to yin and awakening belongs to yang. Calm sleeping (yin) can be divided into deep sleep (yang within yin) and shallow sleep (yin within yin). According to changes of brain waves, sleep can be divided into fast-wave sleep (FWS) and slow-wave sleep (SWS). Fast-wave sleep is relatively shallow and can be easily triggered by external stimuli to produce dream, which belongs to yang within yin. Slow-wave sleep is relatively deep and less susceptible to external stimuli, and thus produce fewer dreams, which belongs to yin within yin. Yin-yang transformation results in a periodic change of fast wave and slow wave overnight, leading to occurrence of multiple dreams.

b) Dream and yin-yang inward movement of defensive qi

People awakes when defensive qi runs in yang aspect during the day and sleeps when it flows in yin aspect at night. Thus, dream occurs when defensive qi flows in yin aspect. According to amount of yin qi, yin aspect can also be divided into three kinds: greater yin, lesser yin, and reverting yin. Greater yin ranks the first because yin qi is the most abundant, also known as extreme yin within yin; lesser yin ranks the second as amount of yin qi is moderate, known as yin within yin; reverting yin is the last one with relatively least yin qi, known as yang within yin (yang waxes when yin wanes). Therefore, as for movement of defensive qi, dream occurs when defensive qi flows to the phase of yang within yin. At this time, activity of dream is different from self-conscious action when defensive qi runs in yang aspect. It is an involuntary image action occurred during sleep when yin qi wanes to a point and cannot constrain yang qi.

c) Dream and yin-yang movement of Shen and ethereal soul

Dynamics of Shen in the day belongs to yang and stability of Shen at night belongs to yin. To go further, ethereal soul following stable Shen and producing no dreams belongs to yin within yin; ethereal soul following dynamic Shen and producing dreams belongs to yang within yin.

3) Yin, yang, and image of dream

Image of dream refers to scenes in dream, also known as dreamscape. There are many factors that affect image of dream, including natural yin-yang changes such as seasons, temperature, and weather, emotional yin-yang changes such as happiness, anger, sorrow, and anxiety, and physiological yin-yang changes like hunger and satiety.

TCM believes that image of dream reflects yin-yang change of viscera, bowels, qi, and blood. When viscera, bowels, qi, and blood are in balance and nutrient qi and defensive qi flow well, sleep and awakening are in an orderly cycle and produce "positive dreams," which are forgotten after people wake up. On the contrary, if yin and yang are imbalanced, viscera, bowels, qi and blood are in disorder, and nutrient qi and defensive qi flows abnormally, "diseased dream" may be produced. Image of dream is closely related to yin-yang imbalance, most of which have characteristics similar to nature and location of disease. For details, please refer to *Miraculous Pivot, Chapter Evil Qi Producing Dream*. Especially in early stage of disease, when people are still unaware of illness in awakening state, they tend to have nightmares, which is often a bad omen, known as "nightmare presaging illness." This image of dream has clinical significance for early diagnosis.

1.5.9 *Theory of Personality and Constitution*

Under the guidance of "unity of form and Shen," theory of personality and constitution emphasizes a close relationship between the two elements mentioned in the title. It not only expounds material basis of personality and constitution from both innate and acquired aspects, but also introduces people of "five yin-yang patterns" and "twenty-five yin-yang types," which are classified in *The Inner Canon of the Yellow Emperor* according to yin, yang, and five elements. Thus, the theory is an indigenous Chinese doctrine with a strong characteristic of traditional Chinese culture. In addition, Xue and Yang launched "*Five-Pattern Personality Inventory*" based on theory of "five yin-yang patterns" in *The Inner Canon of the Yellow Emperor*. It is China's first self-developed psychological measurement tool in line with our national conditions.

LECTURE 2

Grasping the Essentials

Heart Controlling Shen and Mental Development

LECTURER: QU LIFANG

Introduction to the speaker:

Qu Lifang is a professor of Shanghai University of Traditional Chinese Medicine and visiting professor of School of Chinese Medicine, the University of Hong Kong. She is also a chief editor of *Mental Diseases of Traditional Chinese Medicine, Anecdotes of Traditional Chinese Medicine,* and *Selected Case Records of Mental and Psychological Disorders from Past Masters.* Qu has lectured on TCM at University of Sydney, the University of Hong Kong, the University of Malta, University of Eastern Finland, International Medical University of Malaysia, and regions such as Germany and Thailand. She has published more than 60 papers in professional journals at home and abroad. Her clinical expertise is in treatment of mental and emotional disorders using a combination of Chinese medicinal, acupuncture and psychotherapy.

R apid development of modern Western psychology and its quick migration to the East has not only contributed to rapid growth of modern Chinese psychology, but also awakened Chinese people to new understanding and exploration of TCM and local psychology.

Theoretical system of TCM psychology originated from *The Inner Canon of the Yellow Emperor*. Its principles have many similarities with those of modern psychology. TCM believes that "Heart resides the Mind and controls Shen." TCM psychology focuses on and studies Heart Shen, and divides it into three kinds according to different stages and functions of newborn individual development: original Shen, innate Shen, and acquired Shen. These three have important impacts on mental growth and health.

The lecture will mainly expound the cognitive development from Heart "regulating things" to "dealing with matters" in *The Inner Canon of the Yellow Emperor, Divine Pivot, Chapter Original Shen*. It will also present psychological significance of "Heart Controlling Shen" in mental growth and health in *The Inner Canon of the Yellow Emperor, Basic Questions, Chapter Ling Lan*. Besides, the lecture will discuss their relationship and influence, and suggest that psychological problems are more or less related to abnormal function of Heart in cognitive process of "regulating things" and "dealing with matters." To prevent mental illness from starting with Heart "regulating things" at birth, we should pay attention to essential influence exerted by "Heart controlling Shen" on "educating and nurturing." Therefrom, one can have sound mind and personality to "tackle things with wisdom" when he reaches adulthood. In treatment, self-cultivation of Heart Shen is encouraged.

2.1 Introduction

"Heart controlling Shen" is a TCM psychological proposition from *The Inner Canon of the Yellow Emperor*. TCM believes that Heart resides the Mind and controls Shen. Thus, Heart Shen is the core of research in TCM psychology. Heart opens into the tongue. Shen rules body and body houses Shen. Through observation of speech and behavior, doctors can speculate about mental activities and motivations in a critical manner, identify problems and give targeted psychological treatment.

Gui Gu Zi, First Chapter Opening and Closing says, "By observing yin-yang changes, one can make judgements, further understand existence and demise, predict beginning and end in process, comprehend rules of human's psychological changes, reveal signs of change, and thus grasp key to development of all things." "Comprehending rules of human's psychological changes" shows that the ancients had already studied psychological phenomena and it has been applied in military psychological warfare. To have a thorough understanding of "Heart Shen" in TCM.

2.2 Concept of Shen

Traditional Chinese Medicine (TCM) is the main carrier and inheritor of traditional Chinese culture that has been continuous for the last 5,000 years. TCM psychology is based on *The Inner Canon of the Yellow Emperor*, military psychology on *Gui Gu Zi*, and local Chinese psychology on Confucianism. *Book of Changes*, the head of canons, establishes the philosophical outlook of ancient China and has influenced Chinese culture and TCM for thousands of years. Philosophy determines thought and thought controls mental activities. Psychological phenomena are essentially cultural phenomena. Concept of "Shen" in traditional Chinese culture is almost identical to that in TCM psychology.

Origin of Chinese Characters says, "Heaven and Shen are producers of everything." Heaven above is formless as a circle, referring to space and nature; Shen refers to magic natural force that is mighty and invisible. In the oracle bone script of character "Shen (神)," its right side represents a person kneeling and bending in worship, while the left side represents an offering table and offerings, with nothing in front of the table. This is similar to forms and actions of today's Tibetan lamas piling up prayer flags, and people in Inner Mongolia making OBOOs to pay homage to gods of mountains, waters and grasslands. All of these show awe to natural divine forces that create and control everything.

Book of Changes, Chapter General Overview says, "Both Shen and change have no form." In ancient times, there is a saying that "heaven is round while earth is quadrate," which is actually a philosophical concept. Heaven is round without form, while earth is quadrate with form. As Tai Chi is invisible without form, it is drawn as circle. "Shen has no form" means that Shen has no shape but can measure entity. The philosophical concept of *Book of Changes* is trinity of Tao (way), Xiang (image) and Qi (measurement). "Abstract and spiritual things is called Tao; concrete and material things is called Qi." "Tao is yin and yang." "Seeing is Xiang and forming is Qi."

The character "器(Qi)" is made up of four squares on top and bottom, with each one representing form. Understanding and study on Qi mainly focuses on validation and quantification of tangible objects. While modern science (including Western medicine) mainly conducts quantitative research on tangible entities at Qi level, TCM psychology studies psychological phenomena at Xiang level. Only by understanding epistemology of trinity in Tao, Xiang and Qi in *Book of Changes* can one understand yin-yang theory and visceral manifestation theory, and thus TCM psychological principles.

The Inner Canon of the Yellow Emperor, Basic Questions, Chapter Origin of Universe writes, "Shen is unpredictability of yin and yang. The ability to flexibly apply principles of Shen without being limited to a particular method is called holiness." From the morphological structure of the oracle bone script "Shen (神)," it is clear that original meaning of Shen is a ritual and psychological act of worshipping natural divine forces. *The Inner Canon of the Yellow Emperor, Basic Questions, Chapter Preserving Life* writes, "Tao comes and goes alone, without demons and gods."

"Shen" creates everything. It is mysterious, omnipotent, omnipresent, and does not rely on will and thought of human. As Shen is far above control of man, people have a supreme reverence for natural divine forces and make a series of worship acts, such as worshipping mountain god when living near a mountain, worshipping river god when living near water, worshipping sea god when sailing, and worshipping earth god when farming, etc. This is fundamentally different from concrete image of God recreated by people with ulterior motives or with concrete cognitive abilities only, which is personalization of natural divine forces.

Man is created by natural forces. Life phenomenon is one of natural phenomena and vitality is a special manifestation of natural forces. As heaven Shen creates human Shen, concept of Shen is introduced into TCM. *The Inner Canon of the Yellow Emperor, Basic Questions, Chapter Profound Discourses* says, "Changes in human body and Shen correspond to changes in nature."

Understanding of Shen in ancient Chinese medicine is similar to that in indigenous Chinese religion, Taoism. *The Inner Canon of the Yellow Emperor, Basic Questions, Chapter Acupuncture Methods* clearly states, "Acupuncture does not merely treat diseases. It has significance of preserving, nourishing, and cultivating genuine qi. The way to cultivate and harmonize Shen and qi lies in persistence. It is important to nourish Shen and qi and to consolidate the fundamentals. When essence and qi are not dissipated, Shen will guard inside and thus preserve genuine qi. Otherwise, one cannot reach genuine state, in which Shen guard heaven qi and guide it back to original qi, known as returning to ancestors." "Shen guarding inside" and "returning to ancestors" relate to religion, which has its origins in man's quest for the ultimate in life and is inseparable from psychology. Psychology of returning to ancestors is an important part of TCM psychology.

2.3 Classification of Shen

Nearly half of contents in *The Inner Canon of the Yellow Emperor* deals with or relates to Shen. And its connotation has been further developed by successive generations of doctors. In TCM, Shen starts from foundation of life, and is divided into three kinds with development of an individual's life: original Shen, innate Shen, and acquired Shen. All three are closely related to Heart controlling Shen, mental growth and health.

2.3.1 Original Shen

Original Shen derives from *The Inner Canon of the Yellow Emperor, Volume Miraculous Pivot, Chapter Original Shen. Origin of Chinese Characters* says, "Origin (Root) is what beneath the tree." From the evolution of Chinese character 本(ben, root), it can be seen that the middle thick part and the horizontal stroke is root, which means the same as "source" and "origin." Similarly, the three dots in middle of the oracle bone script and the "T" in middle of Chinese Bronze Inscriptions refer to "source" and "origin." *Origin of Chinese Characters* says, "Source is where spring gushes." "Origin is where things accumulate." Thus, root and nature of life lie in original Shen, which hides itself in the dark.

 The Inner Canon of the Yellow Emperor mentions "Shen" for many times. Once it says, "One who gains Shen is healthy while one who does not is in danger of death." *The Inner Canon of the Yellow Emperor, Basic Questions, Chapter Five Circuits* says, "Shen roots inside and qi outside. Human body cannot function when either Shen or qi stops working." *The Inner Canon of the Yellow Emperor, Volume Miraculous Pivot, Chapter Original Shen* writes, "Essence accompanies birth. Spirit is the fusion of yin essence and yang essence." Thus, birth of new life and the new life itself is Shen. This is the "humanistic" concept of TCM psychology: every living individual is considered Shen. The reason why two essences can be fused into new life is that there is Shen in them. Without Shen, two essences cannot be fused, that is, sperm and egg cannot combine. Male is sterile and female is infertile, and thus new life cannot be produced. "Spirit is the fusion of yin essence and yang essence" demonstrates TCM view on "essence and Shen," which is similar to "unity of form and Shen" in Confucianism, Buddhism, and Taoism.

 Undoubtedly, human beings have acquired complex physical and psychological structures in the course of evolution. *The Inner Canon of the Yellow Emperor, Volume Miraculous Pivot, Chapter Five Colors* says, "Shen is accumulated in Heart to know the past and present." Original Shen carries, deposits, and refines all kinds of life information humans have acquired since beginning of evolution, including various unforgettable experiences and instincts of survival. Miscellaneous magical abilities of human beings are all related to Shen, including learning, comprehension, memory, imagination, creativity, thinking, cognition, endurance, willpower, self-control, self-knowledge, intelligence quotient, emotional quotient, as well as teachability, tendency of personality formation, and possibility of personality establishment, etc. Confucius said, "Food and sex is human's nature." This is an outreach of function of original Shen.

 The hidden original Shen is basis for prototype of analytic psychology, support for psychological activities, foundation of personality formation and development, and source of internal motivation. As original Shen belongs to state of selflessness or superego, or to level of superconscious aspect or unconsciousness, it is difficult for general consciousness of human beings to perceive, and is therefore ignored by modern scientific psychology. Study of human psychology in modern psychology is mostly intergenerational, that is, it explores root of psychological problems from visitor's generation to the last second or third generations at most, neglecting deep roots of psychological problems from life chain.

2.3.2 Innate Shen

Innate Shen is also known as brain Shen. In the Ming Dynasty, Li Shizhen's *Compendium of Materia Medica, Chapter Xin Yi* says, "Brain is the palace for innate Shen." *The Inner Canon of the Yellow Emperor, Volume Miraculous Pivot, Chapter Original Shen* writes, "Spirit is the fusion of yin essence and yang essence." Before two essences are fused, Shen contained in each of them is original Shen. Thereafter, new life is born. The magical force that initiates and drives development of new life is innate Shen.

Origin of Chinese Characters says, "Innate Shen is the origin of qi." Qi produces images and images can be seen by people. From ancient times to the present, shape of character "元" (yuan) has changed, but its meaning remains the same. The upper horizontal stroke represents heaven and the second represents earth. The left-handed stoke refers to left root going down first, and the right-handed vertical curved hook refers to right root growing down. Only when roots are stable and vitality is flourishing can innate Shen be noticed. Therefore, function of innate Shen is also difficult for general consciousness of human beings to be aware. Fetus in mother's womb has neither consciousness nor memory.

Original Shen is source of innate Shen, and innate Shen is stream of original Shen. Original Shen is static and lurks in life, while innate Shen is dynamic and thrives in life. These two are sequential but inseparable. At the beginning of life, embryonic tissues and organs continue growing, which is inevitably accompanied by development of original Shen and innate Shen. *The Inner Canon of the Yellow Emperor, Volume Miraculous Pivot, Chapter Natural Life Span* writes, "Yellow Emperor asks Qi Bo what lays foundation for and guards the formation of life, and what birth and death depends on. Qi Bo answers that mother is the foundation and father the guard. Shen determines one's birth and death." The discourse emphasizes the dominant role of original Shen and innate Shen in birth of life.

Life is a highly sophisticated and self-organizing process. *The Inner Canon of the Yellow Emperor, Volume Miraculous Pivot, Chapter Meridian Vessels* states, "In birth of human being, essence is produced first, and then brain and marrow are generated.

Bones construct skeleton, and vessels carry nutrients." At the beginning of life, innate essences from parents first satisfy needs of brain and marrow formation to nourish innate Shen and thus help brain grow normally. Brain, the palace for innate Shen, is full of essence. When brain Shen is bright, people is born with abundant energy, clear hearing, good eyesight, acute thinking, and agile action. Otherwise, if innate essence cannot nurture brain, resulting in essence deficiency, weakness, decline and depletion, it will have an impact on innate brain growth or acquired brain degeneration. The former can lead to congenital stupidity, while the latter can lead to Alzheimer's disease, which belongs to category of "brain Shen lacking brightness." *The Inner Canon of the Yellow Emperor, Basic Questions, Chapter Profound Discourse on Pulse* says, "Head is house of intelligence, which can observe, distinguish, and judge things." This is the theoretical basis for "brain controlling Shen."

Innate Shen is the initiating force activating new life, the magic power exciting original Shen to show up, and the driving force promoting the entire life process. All ways are integrated into one basic principle, so are things. All living things begin from germination of a seed, showing their roots and nature from inside to outside. It must be the same as every human life. Innate Shen triggered original Shen to reveal physical and psychological qualities of race, family, and individual as life processes. A person's intelligence quotient (IQ), physical height, facial appearance, and susceptibility to disease, etc., are closely related to genetic factors at birth. Similarly, a person's IQ, EQ, psychological traits, and personality types, etc. are also inevitably influenced by innate factors. This is described in detail in *The Inner Canon of the Yellow Emperor, Basic Questions, Chapter Twenty-five yin-yang Types of Human*.

In the long chain of human evolution and development, every individual only shortly exists as a small ring. One's form and Shen not only inherit ancestors' traits, but also integrated their own qualities in life process. Each generation is not only a copy of previous one, but also an improved result under influence of acquired environment, and an innovative product after evolution. It is passed down from generation to generation. In terms of physical form, innate Shen controls many instinctive activities such as breath, heartbeat, metabolism, birth, growth, strength, oldness, death and innate desires, which cannot be acquired through learning, but evolution instead. In terms of spirit, innate Shen is related to unconsciousness, intuition, extra sensory perception, etc. It is source of internal motivation for psychological activities.

2.3.3 Acquired Shen

Acquired Shen is also known as Heart Shen. It is a collective concept composed of five visceral Shen: Heart Shen (the innate Shen residing in Heart), ethereal soul of Liver, corporeal soul of Lung, thought of Spleen, and will of Kidney. Acquired Shen leads process of acquired cognitive development, in which Heart Shen is the dominator.

The Inner Canon of the Yellow Emperor, Volume Miraculous Pivot, Chapter Natural Life Span says, "Yellow Emperor asks what is Shen. Qi Bo answers that when qi and blood are harmonized, nutrient qi and defensive qi are unified. Five viscera are flourished and Heart resides Shen and qi. Ethereal soul and corporeal soul are produced and thus human beings exist." There are three meanings in the discourse. First, human is Shen. Second, "Heart (Shen) resides (innate) Shen and qi. Ethereal soul (of Liver) and corporeal soul (of Lung) are produced." Growth of body is process of innate Shen residing in Heart and becoming Heart Shen. Third, only when Shen, ethereal soul, and corporeal soul are all generated can human being exists. One who does not gain Shen is in danger of death. A person dies without original Shen and lives in a coma or vegetative state without acquired Shen but innate Shen. Only when acquired Shen exists can one have psychological activities such as consciousness, thinking, emotion, spirit, etc. Acquired Shen is obtained after birth, while original Shen is inherent. Innate Shen lies between two. There is an order among the three, that is, a relationship of source and stream, which should not be confused. In addition, the reason why the discourse does not mention will and thought is that these two are acquired gradually with cognitive development after birth. It shows the ancients' precise and meticulous observation of psychological development.

From the above, TCM psychology believes that human psychological traits are influenced by three factors in formation and development. The first one is inborn accumulation during evolution of original Shen, which is genetically inherited and passed down from generation to generation. The second is activation of innate Shen. It helps guide and even sometimes dominates psychological development and personality formation. It is source of internal motivation and instinctive desire. The third is influence of acquired Shen on psychological growth through cognition to the external world after birth, which is subject of Heart controlling Shen, cultivating Heart Shen, mental growth, psychological health, and psychotherapy. Original Shen is unconscious or superconscious. Innate Shen is unconscious when connected with original Shen deep inside, and is subconscious when connected with acquired Shen outside. Acquired Shen is conscious when one is awake and uses five senses and orifices. When one sleeps, acquired Shen returns to five viscera and remains subconscious, such as conscious activities during sleep. In Sigmund Freud's *The Interpretation of Dreams*, it writes, "Dream is kind of consciousness, with subconscious floating up to conscious level. It is an avenue to subconscious and a window into the inner world." In fact, words and actions in dream are also a kind of psychological phenomenon.

What each of us can perceive is only the superficial conscious activity controlled by acquired Shen. We cannot perceive and control the deep subconscious and unconscious part. Therefore, I am I, or I am not; I know myself, or I do not. The relationship among the three is shown in Figure 2-1.

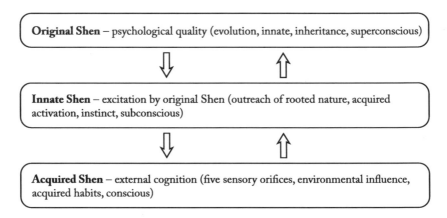

Figure 2-1 Relationship among original Shen, innate Shen, and acquired Shen

Each person's psychological traits and personality formation must be continually influenced by three factors: rooted nature of original Shen, activation and outreach of innate Shen, and cultivation of acquired Shen. As an old saying goes, one can never harvest beans by planting melons. In life process, physical and psychological traits, which are originated from rooted nature inside sperm and the egg, are simultaneously revealed with development of form and Shen, and are passed down from generation to generation like seeds sprouting and blossoming. *The Inner Canon of the Yellow Emperor, Basic Questions, Chapter Acupoints* says, "A sage is easy to talk with, like a good horse is easy to ride on." *The Inner Canon of the Yellow Emperor, Volume Miraculous Pivot, Chapter Confusion* says, "Heart and Shen have their own likes and dislikes." Therefore, people have instinctive orientation for goodness and badness, and inherent differences in teachability.

2.3.4 "Regulating Things," "Dealing with Matters," and Mental Growth

Heart "regulating things" and "dealing with matters" describe cognitive development in TCM of Chinese medicine. *The Inner Canon of the Yellow Emperor, Volume Miraculous Pivot, Chapter Original Shen* says, "… Heart regulates things. Thought is what heart memorizes, and will is where thought is stored. Consideration is to accumulate thoughts and make change. Contemplation is to expand consideration. Wisdom is to deal with matters based on contemplation." "Regulating things" and "dealing with matters" summarize cognitive development process in TCM psychology, and formation and mental development of "thought" and "will." The whole process from birth to death is related to Heart controlling Shen and cultivation of Shen. Understanding development of "regulating things" and "dealing with matters" can provide insight into root and crux of psychological problems, making psychotherapy more targeted and effective.

(1) Heart Shen regulating things: information perception

"Heart regulates things." It means that Heart Shen dominates five senses and orifices to receive various sensory stimuli and information. There are two sources of information that Heart Shen can perceive and receive: inside the body and outside the body. Thus, there are also two ways and processes for Heart Shen "regulating things." Inside-the-body source, for one thing, originates from stimulation of original Shen and innate Shen, such as phenomenon of consciousness returning to ancestors. For another, it comes from physiological and pathological states inside, such as sense of hunger and thirst, feeling of urination and defecation, etc. Outside-the-body source originates from external stimuli. Both sources interact with each other.

1) Regulating things outside and perceiving information through orifices
Process of "regulating things" outside is guided by heart Shen and coordinated by five viscera Shen (spirit, ethereal soul, corporeal soul, thought, will), five senses (eyes, ears, nose, tongue, mouth), and five constituents (sinew, vessel, muscle, skin, bone). From the first time a baby opens his eyes to see the world, he stays in a continuous process of "regulating things," including receiving all kinds of information, being taught by words and actions, learning, and working, etc.

The process involves visual information received and transmitted by Liver, ethereal soul and eyes; information of kinesiology and balance information received and transmitted by Liver and sinew (Liver opens into the eyes, stores ethereal soul and controls sinews); tactile, perceptual and olfactory information received and transmitted by Lung, nose and skin (Lung opens into the nose, controls the skin, manifests in the body hair, and stores corporeal soul); verbal information expressed and transmitted by Heart, spirit and tongue (Heart opens into the tongue, governs blood and vessels, resides spirit, and blood houses spirit); gustatory information and deep perceptual information received and transmitted by Spleen, thought and mouth (Spleen opens into the mouth, controls the muscle, and resides thought); auditory information received and transmitted by Kidney, will, and ears (Kidney opens into the ears, controls the bone, and resides will). All those information is collected to Heart Shen. Five senses are highly generalized as magic orifices, whose perceptual function is an important part in function of acquired Shen. Acquired Shen is the main participant in cognition, but is not exactly the same as Heart Shen. Without support of ethereal soul, corporeal soul, thought, and will, Heart Shen cannot complete cognitive process, as shown in Figure 2-2.

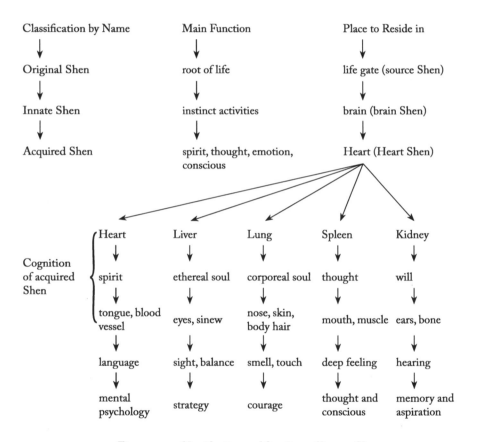

Figure 2-2 *Classification and functions of human Shen*

"Heart regulates things." On one hand, it emphasizes that Heart (Shen) dominates fives senses perceiving external objects. One the other hand, it states that perception of five senses occurs only with participation of Heart (Shen). Distracted mind, scattered or confused Shen, loss of Shen, and Shen not acting on five senses can all prevent Heart Shen from "regulating things."

Gui Gu Zi, Chapter Cultivating Spirit says, "Information is perceived through orifices." Perceiving information generally refers to function of cognition. Orifices refer to sensory apertures, such as eyes, ears, nose, tongue, mouth, external genitalia, anus, skin and sweat pores. Orifices lying on the surface indicate that human's perception and cognition of external information are coordinated and participated by various senses. *Gui Gu Zi, Chapter Power* says, "Ears and eyes are assistants of Heart." Zhang Jiebin also emphasized that eyes and ears assist Heart Shen to perform function of "regulating things." His *Classified Classic, Chapter Fluid and Humor* says, "Heart controls what ears hear and what eyes see." Process of "regulating things" can be either a positive course of purifying and cultivating Heart Shen, or a negative one of staining and alienating Heart Shen. As the saying goes, "A person's future can be figured out from his childhood." This is somewhat similar to doctrine of "life script" in Western psychology. In ancient fetal and early childhood education, it says, "Eyes and ears should not perceive evil information." It emphasizes that functions of five senses need to be dominated by noble-minded and virtuous Heart Shen, which is the same as "gentleman does not look at and carries out what is contrary to propriety" in Confucianism.

2) Regulating things outside and residing in Heart

Five viscera Shen, including spirit, ethereal soul, corporeal soul, thought, and will, is called Shen for short. It functions on five senses and orifices outside, and resides in Heart, Liver, Lungs, Spleen, and Kidneys inside. Shen also guides perception of miscellaneous physiological and pathological information in the body, such as various instinctive desires, appetite, sexual desire and other physiological needs, as well as hunger, thirst, pain, urination and defecation, and other physiological and pathological information.

Another special form of "regulating things" is dream. Image of dream can reflect both physical and psychological conditions. *The Inner Canon of the Yellow Emperor* expounds on principle of dream and describes symbolic meaning of dream in detail. When dream appears during sleep, it is the time when form and Shen are united, yin and yang are balanced, five Shen is coordinated, and body and mind are regulated. In the Ming Dynasty, Zhang Jiebin (1563–1640) writes in his *Classified Classic, Chapter Sleep* that "dream is created by Heart." For one thing, dream is part of "Heart regulating things." For another, dream is related to psychological state. There are three sources of dream. First, dream is caused by external stimuli. What is thought in the day may appear in dream at night. Second, dream comes from struggle between healthy qi and pathogenic qi, disturbing five viscera Shen and hindering quiet residence, which may be an omen of illness. Extreme emotions, unpeaceful state of mind, and psychological imbalance can also lead to dream. Thirdly, "subconscious floating up to conscious level" may be a phenomenon of consciousness returning to its ancestors, in which the evolutionary survival experiences accumulated in original Shen are activated. Therefore, throughout the ages, dream interpretation has been an important means of exploring people's inner world and applying psychotherapy.

(2) HEART MEMORIZING: INFORMATION PROCESSING

"Thought is what heart memorizes." This is the first step of acquiring consciousness in cognition, that is, to process and analyze things. Information processing of "Heart memorizing" is summarized as "thought" in *The Inner Canon of the Yellow Emperor, Volume Miraculous Pivot, Chapter Original Shen*. Zhang Jiebin's *Classified Classic, Volume Viscera Manifestation, Chapter Original Shen* says, "Thought is an undetermined idea generated in Heart." Thought is a process of acquiring consciousness and thought dominated by Heart Shen and Spleen, often accompanied by "consciousness," "image," and "ideas." It is generated from mind.

Process of consciousness can be Heart Shen processing, judging, analyzing, synthesizing, generalizing, and finally coming to relevant conclusions based on past or current knowledge and experience on things let grow, i.e., various information perceived and transmitted by five senses and five constituents. It can also be recalling, replaying, reenacting events in the past or combining thoughts to make a judgment about the present situation. This process takes place at level of consciousness, which is a higher level of cognition. It is similar to "mind" of six consciousness (eyes, ears, nose, tongue, body, and mind) in Buddhism, and similar to thinking activity in the present cognitive system. According to Sigmund Freud, "What can be conscious to us must be recognized by the second mental step... Consciousness is a special kind of mental act, which is the product processed from materials of other sources by senses." "The second mental step" exactly refers to "thought is what heart memorizes," process of acquiring consciousness.

As "thought" includes such things as consciousness, ideas, intentions, meanings, images, moods, and so on, "thought is what heart memorizes" also provides an important method for psychotherapy – scene reproduction, also known as thinking therapy in TCM. "Imagery communication therapy," created by Chinese psychologist Zhu Jianjun, is a local Chinese psychotherapy technique that has been recognized worldwide as effective. Psychologists use imagery to recreate "what one memorizes" at level of consciousness, combining role reversal, empathy, untying mental knots, explaining confusion, releasing worries, and expelling demons inside, to realize psychotherapy. Psychological process described in "what one memorizes" can be present or past progressive. Unforgettable spiritual experiences can exist beyond time and space, and have a lasting impact on psychological activity. Therefore, "what one memorizes" naturally becomes an important and effective way for psychologists to understand psychological phenomena and treat mental illness.

"Heart memorizing" can be a single learning process, or a lifelong one. Heart "regulating things" is an immediate process of sense perception, only superficial understanding or acceptance of knowledge. But "Heart memorizing" is deep thinking and processing at the level of consciousness, transforming knowledge into wise "Heart comprehension." This is what *The Analects of Confucius* says, "Isn't it pleasure to constantly review what has been learnt?"

(3) THOUGHT BEING STORED: MEMORY STORAGE

"Will is where thought is stored." It refers to memory, that is, process of storing consciousness, ideas, image derived from previous thinking in Kidney with the participation of Heart (Shen) and Kidney (will). The original meaning of "will" is memory. From "thought" to "will," it is both a processing and memory course, as well as a process of coming to a decision and aspiration after repeated thinking and contemplation.

We gradually obtained "thought" and "will" during the process, including growth and maturity of ideological awareness and acquisition and stability of willpower. Thought and will is kind of perseverance, a relatively unchanging goal in life, a spirit of persistence. Thought and will is relatively stable and not easily changed. TCM believes that will of Kidney contains human's intelligence, aspiration, memory and other abilities. "Will" is closely related to one's Kidney essence. When one is young and has abundant kidney essence and flouring Kidney qi, he can establish great ambition. Sufficient Kidney essence and qi contribute to strong storage ability and good memory. Thus, one should study as early as possible.

"Regulating things," "Heart memorizing," and "thought being stored" represents environment perception and three processes of information reception, preliminary processing, and memory storage, which are input-oriented processes of consciousness. These three are complementary, highly coordinated and instantaneous. For example, in *The Inner Canon of the Yellow Emperor, Volume Miraculous Pivot, Chapter Original Shen*, it says, "Ethereal soul follows Spirit forward and backward." When Liver and ethereal soul (eyes) see things, Heart Shen "regulates things" and "memorizes" at the same time to make immediate judgment whether it is known or unknown. If Shen and ethereal soul do not follow each other, known as "Shen distracted" or "ethereal soul lost," Heart Shen cannot "regulate things" normally, interrupting cognitive processes of perception, cognition, consciousness, thinking, judgment, storage, etc. If learning process is a complete one, from "regulating things" to "Heart memorizing" and "thought being stored," knowledge will be grasped more firmly and longer. All of these should be based on "Heart controlling Shen." Difference between "straight A students" and "study slackers" also lies in the process.

(4) Accumulating thoughts and making change: deep thinking

"Consideration is to accumulate thoughts and make change." It represents a process of maturing and perfecting the consciousness, a process of constantly adjusting "will" to the environment, a process of accumulating knowledge and experience, and improving one's ability to think. However, compared with thought in "thought is what heart memorizes," here it refers to deeper and higher level of consideration. As Zhang Jiebin wrote in *Classified Classic, Volume Viscera Manifestation*, "Will is determined thought." As "memory" is a simple, primary judgment of external information, thought based on "will" is deep processing of internal accumulated knowledge. Quantitative change leads to qualitative one. Finally, with sublimated knowledge, growing wisdom, and enlightened mind, one can achieve purpose of mental growth.

(5) Expanding consideration: contemplation

"Contemplation is to expand consideration." It refers to process of repeatedly pondering and contemplating realization of an ambition or ideal for the long term. "Contemplation" and "expand" here has the meaning of planning and strategizing. *On Extinction of Soul* suggests that "shallow thinking is knowledge, while deep one is contemplation." Sayings such as "tranquility in mind leads to big ambition," "great aspirations trigger strategy," and "think before one leaps" are all related to contemplation. Establishment of aspirations and realization of ideals should be based on "Heart controlling Shen." Otherwise, delusions or paranoia will be induced, or even develop into paranoia, rhapsody or idiot scholars.

(6) "Dealing with matters" based on contemplation: knowledge producing intelligence

"Wisdom is to deal with matters based on contemplation." This is sign of mental maturity. "Dealing with matters" is an ability to analyze and deal with various issues with wisdom. Yang Shangshan (585–670) wrote in Great Simplicity of *The Inner Canon of the Yellow Emperor*, "Wisdom is used by Shen. It means to deal with matters based on contemplation." Thought and contemplation produce wisdom. Therefore, thought, contemplation and wisdom are process of accumulating knowledge and sublimating it from quantity to quality, as well as process of internalizing all kinds of knowledge and applying it flexibly. Three stages of thought, contemplation, and wisdom are process of sublimating knowledge and gaining ability to "deal with things" after "regulating things."

Cognitive development from "regulating things" to "dealing with matters" concisely summarizes whole process of human mental development in TCM psychology. From birth to death, it can be basically generalized into three stages.

1) Cognition: "Regulating things"

It is process of perceiving and receiving external information by senses such as eyes, ears, nose, tongue, and body, which accompanies one's whole life from the first sight of the world at birth to closing eyes and leaving the world. Five senses and orifices influence cultivation and brightness of Shen through stimulation of external environment and natural reactions.

2) Processing: "Heart memorizing" and "thought being stored"

It is course of processing and storing information after thought at level of "consciousness." Telling right from wrong and learning from mistakes can be a learning process of a lesson, an event, a stage, or mental growth of a craft, a job, a generation, or even a lifetime. Most importantly, Heart controlling Shen must always accompany these processes.

3) Wisdom production: "accumulating thoughts, making change, expanding consideration, and thus dealing with matters"

It is process of deep processing, re-outputting, and re-applying knowledge, as well as process of Heart Shen continuously getting cultivated and becoming brighter. Knowledge, intelligence quotient (IQ), and emotional quotient (EQ) are neutral in nature. They can only function properly when being used correctly under the circumstance of "Heart controlling Shen."

These three processes basically represent process of acquiring knowledge after birth. Any of these processes must be ruled by Heart Shen, guided by "Heart controlling Shen" to achieve goal of "mental growth." If Heart Shen is not bright, one will make mistakes. *The Inner Canon of the Yellow Emperor, Volume Miraculous Pivot, Chapter Five Colors* says, "Shen is accumulated in Heart to know the past and present." It refers to process of acquired Shen obtaining knowledge and accumulating experience. It can be accumulation of one generation, or even more. *Gui Gu Zi, Chapter Cultivating Spirit* says, "When there is desire, will exists and thinks of it. Will is the subordinate of desire. Excess desire can distract Heart and thus weaken will." "If will is settled, Heart is calm, and action cam be proper." "With a strong Heart and determined will, thought is on the right track." *The Inner Canon of the Yellow Emperor, Volume Miraculous Pivot, Chapter Pathogen* says, "Heart is the great master of five viscera and six bowels and houses essence and Shen." As for descendants, they propose "dedicating to realizing will," "tranquility in mind leading to big ambition," and "living a simple life and clarifying one's will." All of these emphasize dominating, leading and guiding role of Heart Shen on ethereal soul, corporeal soul, thought, and will. Heart Shen is responsible for "regulating things" while Heart intellect for "dealing with matters." From "regulating things" to "dealing with matters," it is process of Heart controlling and cultivating Shen. It is not inherent for Heart to control Shen. Heart must be cultivated and corrected to gradually transform Shen from "obscurity" to "brightness." If Heart Shen is not bright enough, it can be confused or stained, causing many psychological problems such as drug addiction and Internet addiction, etc.

The Inner Canon of the Yellow Emperor, Basic Questions, Chapter Formation of Five Viscera says, "Size, smoothness, depth of pulse can be differentiated. Therefrom, manifestation and pitches of five viscera can be deduced and be aware of." Zhang Jiebin explained the discourse as follows, "Manifestation means types of image, like twenty-five yin-yang types of human being. Pitches refer to five notes: jue (Mi) of Liver, zhi (So) of Heart, gong (Do) of Spleen, shang (Re) of Lung, and yu (La) of Kidney." In fact, "manifestation" here is similar to "appearance" of "appearance originating from Heart" in Buddhism. "Pitches" can be sounds accompanying the scene. As is mentioned, manifestation and pitches of five viscera can be aware of. And there are internal and external ways for Heart to memorize and acquire consciousness. Therefore, thinking therapy in TCM uses manifestation and pitches of "Heart memorizing," i.e., scene reproduction, to treat certain psychological diseases. "Mistaking the reflection of a bow for a snake is a successful case."

Process of "regulating things" and "dealing with matters" in TCM psychology reveals that there are two kinds of world that the general human consciousness can perceive. One is perception of external objective world when wide awake. The other is perception of internal subjective world during sleep (and sometimes in coma). The inner world includes scenes, events, emotions, and character activities in dream. A complete cognitive process starts from "Heart (Shen) regulates things" to "thought is what heart memorizes" (acquisition of consciousness), and finally ends in "will is where thought is stored." From this we can see that process of "regulating things" must be remembered clearly if Heart Shen participates and lead the whole course. If Shen of five viscera is in disorder, normal cognitive process of "regulating things" and "dealing with matters" will be disrupted. Thus, subjective and objective worlds seen by the person concerned will be distorted and various strange illusions will appear.

On February 28, 2012, I visited the exhibition "Fantastic Creatures from the British Museum" in Hong Kong. There are many bizarre beasts, such as a fish-bodied human-faced creature, a goat-legged human-bodied creature, and a lion-bodied human-faced creature, as well as many grotesque drawings. The commentaries suggest that these are based on descriptions of what one sees in his dream.

In *The Inner Canon of the Yellow Emperor, Basic Questions, Chapter Genuine Words*, it proposes that five elements (wood, fire, earth, metal, and water) combines with five viscera (Liver, Heart, Spleen, Lung, Kidney), five livestock (chicken, sheep, cow, horse, and pig), five fruits, five vegetables, five colors, and five flavors. If functions of viscera and bowels are out of balance, or if various pathogens interfere with functions of five viscera Shen (spirit, ethereal soul, corporeal soul, thought, and will), it will make function of Heart Shen "regulating things" and "dealing with matters" abnormal. Thus, things combined with five viscera such as livestock, objects, and colors will appear in people's mind, eyes, or image of dreams during sleep. When described after people wake up, these things become fantastic creatures or scenes only seen by "witness." This is one of the reasons explaining hallucinations of psychopaths.

Zhang Jiebin's *Classified Classic, Chapter Dream* says, "Five elements originate from infinity, and dream is created by Heart. Heart is the monarch and houses Shen. When Shen is active in Heart, five viscera Shen responds and acts. Thus, where Heart reaches lies Shen, and where Shen reaches lies Heart. Heart and Shen interact with each other. Emotions or confusion in one's heart can lead to dream because Heart controls Shen.... Soul of Heart reaches wherever it can, and thus dream shows whatever can be seen. Indeed, there can be scenes one fails to describe." Ancient TCM experts summarized psychological problems as interruption of emotions and confusion, showing their profound insights. In a training session for college counselors in Shanghai, a student asked, "I always dream that I am at a crossing and don't know which way to go. What does this imply?" I replied, "You haven't made a final decision about your career." She agreed, "Yes, I'm still on the fence."

2.4 Nurturing Heart Shen with Virtue in Confucianism to Make it Bright

In *The Inner Canon of the Yellow Emperor*, it states several times that "Heart is the organ similar to the monarch and controls Shen and mental activity." "Heart controlling Shen" has thus become the primary and important issue in TCM psychology. TCM believes that either things in the world or human society is a unity of yin and yang. The reason why Heart Shen should be cultivated is that living environment of each individual includes both positive (yang) and negative (yin) aspects. In long history of evolution, human beings have experienced both good times and bad times, have accumulated both positive and negative energies, and have grown both bright and dark sides. In cognitive development of "regulating things" and "dealing with matters," if one wants to transform knowledge into mental growth, healthy psychology and sound personality under the guidance of "Heart controlling Shen," he should intentionally distinguish yin from yang in quality of root and origin, that is, to strengthen and develop positive accumulation, and to weaken and remove negative accumulation.

Taoism, China's indigenous religion, and Buddhism, which was introduced to China from India, have many studies in cultivating Heart Shen for reference. Meanwhile, Confucianism represented by Confucius's "doctrine on man of virtue" has been integrated in Chinese system of educating and nurturing for long. The reason why there are more psychological problems today is that Chinese parents fail to handle relationship between "educating" and "nurturing." They tend to separate these two, prioritize "nurturing," or even abandon both. In fact, "educating" should come first and "nurturing" follows. They are inseparable and should be integrated into one.

(1) HEART CONTROLS SHEN AND SERVES AS MONARCH

The Inner Canon of the Yellow Emperor, Basic Questions, Chapter Acupuncture Methods says, "Heart is the organ similar to the monarch and controls Shen and mental activity. ... Spleen is the organ similar to an official of admonition and provides advice." *The Inner Canon of the Yellow Emperor, Basic Questions, Chapter Ling Lan* says, "Heart is the organ similar to the monarch and controls Shen and mental activity. Lung is the organ similar to the prime minister and is responsible for management and regulation. Liver is the organ similar to a general in the army and is responsible for making strategy. Gallbladder is the organ similar to an official of justice and is responsible for decision. Pericardium is the organ similar to the envoy and controls happiness and joy. Spleen and stomach are organs similar to the granary and are responsible for digestion, absorption and transportation of the five flavors. Large intestine is the organ similar to the official in charge of transportation and is responsible for change and transformation. Small intestine is the organ similar to the official in charge of reception and is responsible for further digestion of foods. Kidney is the organ similar to the official with great power and is responsible for developing methods and skills. Triple energizer is the organ similar to the official in charge of dredging and is responsible for regulating water passage. Bladder is the organ similar to the official in charge of reservoir and is responsible for accumulation and discharge of liquids through qi transformation. These twelve officials constitute human body and interact with each other. When Shen is bright, officials function well and human is in good health. Applying the same principle can attain prosperity for a country. When Shen is confused, officials are in disorder, blocking passage and damaging human body. A country will be in danger and chaos under the same circumstance. Warning!"

Both discourses use metaphor of a ruler governing a country to explain influence of Heart as monarch on other viscera and bowels, and its importance in physical and mental health. Brightness of Heart Shen is the cornerstone of physical and mental health, while confusion of Heart Shen is root of physical and mental illness.

1) Brightness of Heart Shen contributes to longevity

"Heart controlling Shen" in *The Inner Canon of the Yellow Emperor* has three meanings. First, as the monarch, Heart has virtue of gentleman. Second, Heart is ruler of Shen. Shen dominates, controls, and regulates the whole body. Thus, "Heart is the great master of body." Third, Heart Shen must be bright. Heart Shen is like ruler of a nation. A nation cannot survive without a ruler for one day, not to mention a fatuous one; a body cannot live without Heart Shen for one day, not to mention a confused one. "Bright" has multiple meanings, such as knowing things clearly, telling right from wrong, understanding issues explicitly without confusion, and being wise and rational. *The Inner Canon of the Yellow Emperor* highly summarizes the complex psychological phenomena into two aspects: "brightness of Heart Shen" and "confusion of Heart Shen." Whether Heart Shen is bright or not is not only an important indicator of judging an individual's ability to "regulate things" and to "deal with matters," state of psychological health and soundness of personality, but also an important factor in determining whether one suffers from mental, emotional and psychological disorders. All human mental activities and behavior can be discussed under this category.

Everyone's acquired Shen starts from state of obscurity at birth and gradually becomes clear with parents' words and deeds, surrounding environment, various enlightenment education, knowledge education and humanistic education from childhood to adulthood. Change of Heart Shen from obscurity to brightness is a long and complex process of psychological growth, which is closely related to family environment, education level, social and cultural background, psychological formation, level of psychological maturity, psychological correction, psychological sanity and many other psychological factors. When environment is good, acquired Shen is positive, making Heart Shen bright. When Shen is as bright as a mirror, Heart works properly, avoid distractions outside and delusions inside. Brightness of Heart Shen can guide individuals to form correct values of life, in which rational, healthy thinking stays in a dominant position to wisely deal with various successes and setbacks, and thus can help obtain good psychological qualities and form sound personality. Lao Tzu said, "He who knows others is wise, and he who knows himself is bright. He who beat others is powerful, and he who beat himself is strong. He who has a contented mind is well-off. He who sticks to action is ambitious." Therefore, to cultivate Heart Shen, self-knowledge is the first priority. Knowing oneself is valuable, which can contribute to brightness of Heart Shen and longevity of human life.

2) Confusion of Heart Shen leads to officials in disorder

Brightness of Heart Shen is closely related to innate and acquired factors. Buddhism believes that inner world of man is divided into two systems: "original" and "newly edified," namely, "innate" and "acquired." "Innate" refers to an individual's inborn psychological qualities, such as good nature, recklessness, caution, carelessness, and introversion. "Acquired" refers to psychological characteristics that one gradually develops through learning and cultivation, such as thinking twice before acting, being calm and experienced, speaking elegantly, and acting politely. Innate system is more dominated by inborn factors, while acquired one is more influenced by acquired factors. Both two interact with each other and determines degree and scope of brightness of Heart Shen to a certain extent.

In the acquired process of "regulating things" and "dealing with matters," acquired Shen perceives surrounding environment through eyes, ears, nose, tongue, and body. Sight belongs to acquired Shen of eyes, hearing to acquired Shen of ears, smell to acquired Shen of nose, taste to acquired Shen of tongue, sense of skin to acquired Shen of body, and mind to acquired Shen of consciousness. Environment of "regulating things" and "dealing with matters" will have influence on acquired Shen. If one lies down with dogs, he will get up with fleas. A correct, positive, good environment will contribute to brightness of Heart Shen, while a wrong, negative, evil one results in confusion of Heart Shen, which can lead to psychopathology or mental abnormality due to deviations and variations in external world and inner experiences perceived by five senses. This is basis of mental and psychological illness, and is closely related to personality disorder, abnormality, mutation and defects.

Confusion of Heart Shen can lead to a perverted ego and, if circumstances are unfavorable during one's growth, particular social personality patterns may develop. For instance, patients with depression often sees dark side of society and gradually develops an antisocial personality. Patients with hypochondriasis are more suspicious and guarded, and are prone to form delusions of persecution, leading to overreaction and aggressive behavior. On one hand, it can lead to alcoholism, smoking, indulgence and other bad habits, which are consequences of "when Shen is confused, officials are in disorder, blocking passage and damaging human body." On the other hand, staining and confusion of Heart Shen can affect people's spiritual, emotional, and psychological activities, increasing susceptibility of various physical and mental diseases, or mental, emotional, and psychological illness. *Gui Gu Zi, Chapter Reaction* says, "It is incorrect to tackle things without planning and strategy." Lao Tzu advocates "choosing a good place to live" and believes "living in a good place contributes to a kind and benevolent mind and thus satisfying words and deeds."

As two aspects of an important proposition in TCM psychology, "brightness of Heart Shen" and "confusion of Heart Shen" show important relationship among brightness of Heart Shen, mental health and soundness of personality, and among confusion of Heart Shen, psychological disorders and personality defects. These two seem to be individual behavior, but are in fact social one. Level of psychological health and stability of Heart Shen cannot be promoted independently, nor can it be achieved overnight. It is a long way for Heart Shen to develop from obscurity to brightness. As physiological age grows, individual's life experiences are enriched and psychological age matures. With a good social and cultural environment, individual is influenced by positive factors, making one's mind and soul purified, abnormal psychology corrected, and Heart Shen positively strengthened. Thus, Heart Shen can be transformed from small brightness to bigger one. Otherwise, a negative social environment will cause adverse effects, with individual's psychology not corrected in time, mind and soul not purified, and Heart Shen stained and destroyed. Heart Shen will be transformed from brightness to confusion.

3) Cultivating Heart Shen with virtue for lifetime
Everything is changing, and the world is impermanent. In process of "regulating things" and "dealing with matters," Heart Shen continuously faces new environments and issues, and stays in a constant state of being influenced and changing. Thus, Heart Shen should be cultivated for lifetime. Modern education pattern is in general a positive cultivation, but to some extent there are also some bad influences. Effect of materialistic desires and fame can transform brightness into obscurity, such as corruption and degeneration in the real world. However, timely cultivation of Heart Shen can reverse the situation such as forsaking darkness (evil) for light (good), repenting and compensating, etc.

The Inner Canon of the Yellow Emperor, Basic Questions, Chapter Transformation of Qi and Essence says, "Evil cannot penetrate deeply into a world of tranquility and goodness." Despite rich material life in today's society, spiritually man is getting farther away from world of tranquility and goodness. Thus, external world of tranquility and goodness cannot be sought, one has to cultivate his inner mind. *The Inner Canon of the Yellow Emperor, Basic Questions, Chapter Nature* says, "Tranquility and emptiness nurtures genuine qi, making essence and qi guard inside. Then how can illness exist?" This is the highest state of cultivating Heart Shen and nourishing body. "Tranquility" refers to pleasure and happiness; "emptiness" refers to calmness and serenity. When Heart is as pure (calm) as a mirror, free from dust, stain, and confusion, it gets fair and bright, which is the optimal state of Heart Shen. Otherwise, confusion of Heart Shen derives from distracting thoughts and desires, such as improper pursuit of fame and fortune, or abnormal extravagant desire for wealth, etc. All these can make one obsessed with money, power, love, or lust, causing illness, mistakes, or crimes.

In traditional Chinese culture, Confucianism is a model for spiritual cultivation, ethics and morality. The left side of character "儒 (ru, Confucianism)" is character "人 (ren, person)," while its right side is character "需 (xu, need)." It means Confucianism is knowledge necessary as a human being. Virtue of gentleman, represented by Confucianism, is the highest example of noble character, perfect personality and gracious sentiments. Sima Qian's *The Historical Records, Chapter Biography of Confucius* says, "When Confucius was old, he got fond of reading *Book of Changes*. He wrote Tuan, Xi, Xiang, Hexagram, and Words. The book had been broken for several times as Confucius kept studying." Hexagrams in *Book of Changes* have clear norms and methods of practice for virtue of gentleman. I have excerpted several for reference.

a) *Book of Changes, Chapter Qian* says, "As heaven maintains vigor through movements, a gentleman should constantly strive for self-perfection. ... A gentleman is always self-improving and diligent all day long. ... A gentleman accumulates knowledge through learning, argues clearly through discussion, handles things with generosity, and acts with benevolence and justice."

b) *Book of Changes, Chapter Kun* says, "A gentleman should hold the outer world with broad mind."

c) *Book of Changes, Chapter Meng* says, "A gentleman should act decisively to cultivate good morals."

d) *Book of Changes, Chapter Song* says, "A gentleman should think foresight before doing things and eliminate factors that may cause disputes from the beginning."

e) *Book of Changes, Chapter Da You* says, "A gentleman should forbid bad things and promote good things."

f) *Book of Changes, Chapter Qian* says, "A gentleman should maintain a humble attitude to improve his self-cultivation"

g) *Book of Changes, Chapter Sui* says, "A gentleman should behave differently with change of time, work diligently during the day, and rest at night."

h) *Book of Changes, Chapter Gu* says, "A gentleman should help the people and cultivate his own virtues."

i) *Book of Changes, Chapter Yi* says, "A gentleman should speak cautiously and eat in moderation."

j) *Book of Changes, Chapter Da Guo* says, "A gentleman should be strong enough without fear in great adversity, and should not feel depressed even if not recognized by the world."

k) *Book of Changes, Chapter Xian* says, "A gentleman should be humble enough to widely accept others' opinions."

l) *Book of Changes, Chapter Dun* says, "A gentleman should avoid short-sighted people, not hate them, but take them seriously. A gentleman can retreat bravely, while base persons cannot."

m) *Book of Changes, Chapter Da Zhuang* says, "A gentleman should be strict with themselves and not behave improperly beyond rules and laws."

n) *Book of Changes, Chapter Jia Ren* says, "A gentleman should speak based on facts and actively put words into deeds."

o) *Book of Changes, Chapter Sun* says, "A gentleman should suppress anger, greed and desire."

p) *Book of Changes, Chapter Yi* says, "A gentleman should learn from good conduct and correct any mistake in time."

q) *Book of Changes, Chapter Sheng* says, "A gentleman should cultivate his own moral character by conforming to the laws of nature, accumulating small progress to shape a noble and perfect personality."

r) *Book of Changes, Chapter Zhen* says, "A gentleman should consciously cultivate his virtues because of fear."

s) *Book of Changes, Chapter Gen* says, "A gentleman should consider matters within his own authority."

t) *Book of Changes, Chapter Jian* says, "A gentleman should accumulate his own virtues, change old habits to get rid of shortcomings."

u) *Confucius* says, "Do these skills mean too much for a gentleman? Not at all."

As can be seen above, virtue of gentleman is hard to master, not to mention cultivating Heart Shen.

4) Brightness of Heart Shen guarantees smooth passage

a) Concept of "passage"

"Smooth passage" is an important part of "brightness of Heart Shen." It originates from *The Inner Canon of the Yellow Emperor, Basic Questions, Chapter Ling Lan.* "When Shen is confused, officials are in disorder, blocking passage and damaging human body." "Passage" here has three meanings: "channel for Shen and qi to function" proposed by Wang Bing (710–804), "way for Shen and qi to flow," and "pathway for Heart Shen to move and act." People who accept other's advice and make fewer mistakes have smooth passage; those who ignore advice and fail to quit bad habits such as smoking, alcoholism, and Internet addiction suffer from blocked passage. As for some stubborn patients with severe mental illnesses like autism, verbal psychotherapy does not work, resulting in blocked passage as well.

In short, passage is the channel of communication between ethereal soul, corporeal soul, thought, and will ruled by Heart Shen and "orifices perceiving information." *Gui Gu Zi, Chapter Correspondence* says, "Heart is ruler of nine orifices." It indicates that perceptual functions of nine orifices, "regulating things" and "dealing with matters" are ruled and driven by Heart Shen.

b) Construction of passage

Construction of passage synchronizes with growth of form and spirit during embryonic period. From "spirit (initiation of new life) is the fusion (fertilized egg) of yin essence and yang essence (with original Shen involved for sure)" to "in birth of human being, essence is produced first, and then brain and marrow (where innate Shen is housed) are generated," and finally to "five viscera are flourished and Heart (Shen) resides Shen (innate Shen) and qi, with ethereal soul (of Liver) and corporeal soul (of Lung) produced and thus human being exists," growth of form and spirit is always accompanied by formation and development of passage. As form and spirit are three-dimensional, so is passage.

Circuits between Heart Shen and ethereal soul, corporeal soul, thought, and will, between five viscera Shen and five senses and orifices (eyes, ears, nose, tongue, and mouth), between Heart Shen and five senses and orifices all belong to category of passage.

Growth of form and spirit is a process developing from small to large, from inside to outside. Before fetus is born, as it does not contact external world directly and independently, viscera Shen such as spirit, ethereal soul, and corporeal soul mostly reside in five viscera and sometimes in sensory orifices. Passage between Heart Shen and five senses and orifices is not completely established and unblocked. Thus, perceptual ability (prenatal education) of fetus is still driven by instincts of innate Shen and belongs to unconscious natural activities.

c) Training in unblocking passage

After birth, fetus contacts external world independently. Sensory orifices being exposed to various external stimuli is beneficial to establishment and perfection of smooth passage, such as auditory training in sound to ears, visual training in light and color to eyes, sensory and tactile stimulation of skin, hair and orifices by parents' kisses and caresses, etc. *Gui Gu Zi, Chapter Cultivating Spirit* says, "Information is perceived through orifices." Five viscera Shen (spirit, ethereal soul, corporeal soul, thought, and will) residing in five organs must move out to body surface to open orifices, which can serve as acquired Shen thereafter. The reason why infants sleep up to 22 or 23 hours a day is that five viscera Shen still reside in five organs and do not move out to sensory orifices. It is well known that viviparous animals, such as wolves, dogs, lions, and leopards, often "lick their calves." Simple act of a female animal licking her newborn cub, which seems like drying wet body, actually implies parental love of training in unblocking passage. The training aims to move five viscera Shen from inside to sensory orifices outside, to construct and unblock channels of communication, and thus to make sensory and tactile reactions of new generation function normally and acutely, laying the foundation for cognition of Heart Shen "regulating things" and "dealing with matters." The fact that oviparous animal must break out of its shell by itself also implies this meaning. Without establishment and smooth flow of passage, Heart cannot regulate things, interrupting cognitive development and acquisition of ability to deal with matters.

Training in unblocking passage for infants and toddlers is gradual and slow. The postnatal period, especially before age of three months, is the critical period for establishment and training in unblocking passage. Parents should consciously stimulate baby's sensory orifices in sound, light, color, language, touch, eye expression, moving scenery and other aspects. This can help move five viscera Shen from inside to outside and construct passage of effective communication between Shen and orifices.

As newborns do not feel pain, they will remember the first unpleasant experience of injection and cry if receiving another one next time. Infants and toddlers cannot differentiate five flavors, but learn about them through repeated experiences and parents' guidance. This is cognitive development of flavors, known as "Heart regulates things; thought is what heart memorizes, and will is where thought is stored." When experiences and knowledge accumulate to a certain extent, it comes to a superior cognitive phase, known as "consideration is to accumulate thought and make change, contemplation is to expand consideration, and wisdom is to deal with things based on contemplation." Therefore, establishment and smooth flow of passage is prerequisite and guarantee for Heart Shen "regulating things" and "dealing with matters."

d) Blockage of passage

The Inner Canon of the Yellow Emperor, Basic Questions, Chapter Ling Lan, "When Shen is confused, officials are in disorder, blocking passage and damaging human body." "Blocking passage" here mainly refers to blocking channel for Shen and qi to function between Heart Shen and twelve officials, which may also include dysfunction of twelve officials and obstruction of qi, blood, fluid, and so on.

During infancy and early childhood, if there is a lack of psychological care and communication with relatives, and passage is not effectively trained for smoothness in early development, child may suffer from autism. Autistic children cannot realize and complete the cognition process mentioned in *The Inner Canon of the Yellow Emperor, Volume Miraculous Pivot, Chapter Original Shen*. Thus, they have extensive cognition disorders and are unable to communicate with others. Their Shen in five viscera does not establish a normal channel with five orifices, resulting in failure of Heart Shen effectively integrating dispersed perceptual functions. Process of "regulating things" cannot be completed and ability to "deal with matters" cannot be acquired. Since internal and external worlds are not interconnected, autistic children can live in a solitary world, which is a serious case of "blocked passage."

In a natural birth, baby's head and skin are squeezed through obstetric canal and closely contact mother's body, which helps to activate "orifices perceiving information" and establish "smooth passage." Infants born by cesarean section do not undergo this process, which may influence function of orifices and passage.

Life is a natural process. During embryonic period, it is best to let embryo develop naturally with minimal human interference. Artificial application of drugs or other means to promote so-called brain growth and neurological development may lead to an asynchronous, uncoordinated or even separated development of form and Shen, which may be one of the causes of autism in children.

Adults' passage can be blocked if obsessed with various inappropriate desires, such as love, power, money, and sex, or due to obstruction of pathogens, such as phlegm clouding pericardium, blood stasis obstructing pericardium, dampness clouding pericardium, etc. This can lead to various mental, psychological, and emotional illnesses, as well as making mistakes, breaking laws, and suffering diseases. Only when Heart Shen is bright, passage is smooth, and five sensory orifices function well can patients take doctor's advice and think clearly, and thus can various psychotherapy techniques and methods work well. Otherwise, all therapies are of no use. For instance, passage of patient with severe depression is often blocked, leading to disinterest in beauty of food, scenery, music, color, objects, etc. It is difficult to help him get out of depressed state simply with ordinary psychological counseling.

"Shen can control passage," or "Shen can manage form," impelling functions of viscera and bowels to remain normal. When "Shen cannot control form," functions of viscera and bowels cannot get back to normal state, which is related to sequelae. When elaborating serious illnesses and emotional diseases, *The Inner Canon of the Yellow Emperor, Basic Questions, Chapter Decoction* says, "Yellow Emperor asked the reason why treatment does not work when one's body is decaying, with qi and blood exhausted. Qibao replied that it is due to dysfunction of Shen. Yellow Emperor asked for further information and Qi Bo explained that needles and stones are only tools and must be combined with Shen to regulate life activities. Diseases cannot be cured when essence, qi and Heart Shen are floating, and thought and will are in disorder. Furthermore, if one has many bad habits and keeps being sorrowful and worried, his essence and qi will be corrupted and defensive qi and nutrient qi will be depleted. Thus, Shen cannot function and patients cannot recover." Zhang Wanlin (1764–1833) explained the discourse further, "Way of treatment is that acupuncture and medicine attack pathogen, and Shen and qi help take effect. When treatment is applied outside, Shen responds inside and make medicinal move upward or downward. Thus, Shen rules treatment."

e) Training in making passage incline to smoothness

Training in unblocking passage may be unconscious and natural in early stages of infancy and childhood. However, when it comes to stage of learning, children or parents can choose their own path to success according to their own conditions and preferences. This process of training and cultivating special skills or crafts with clear goals can be classified as acquired training in making passage incline to smoothness. Zhang Jiebin's *Classified Classic, Chapter Dream* says, "When Shen is active in Heart, five viscera Shen responds and acts. Thus, where Heart reaches lies Shen, and where Shen reaches lies Heart. Heart and Shen interact with each other." Where Shen goes has magical function. Place where Heart Shen often comes to and resides in contains one's unique skill. Hands of magician, painter, pianist, basketball player, women of embroidery, feet of soccer player, and three fingers of taking the pulse in TCM are all results of training in making passage incline to smoothness.

2.5 Way of Yin and Yang and Enlightening Heart Shen

Enlightening Heart Shen is acquired psychological development. "Enlightening" means brightness of Heart Shen, knowing one's own characteristics, understanding one's own act, and clarifying one's own needs, etc. Man is unity of yin and yang. Yang is positive and yin is negative. Enlightening Heart Shen is to strengthen and develop positive energy accumulated inside, and to weaken and eradicate the negative energy.

In long process of Heart Shen "regulating things" and "dealing with matters," different environments, situations, and influences can make Shen further positive – establishing a healthy mind and a sound personality; they can also make Shen further negative – producing psychological abnormalities and personality disorders. Whether human's mind turns to good or evil is influenced by both innate and acquired factors. For the same events, experiences, or stimuli, some people choose good and grow more positive, while some others choose evil and grow more negative. Chinese philosophy holds that only eggs, not stones, can hatch chicks in appropriate conditions. This reflects understanding of human nature in Chinese culture.

(1) YIN AND YANG ARE PALACE FOR SHEN

Ancient sages have expounded on theory and methods of enlightening Heart Shen. *Gui Gu Zi, Chapter Cultivating Spirit* says, "Way is origin of Shen" and "Way is principle of cultivating Shen." *Book of Changes* says, "Way is yin and yang." Theory of yin and yang is not only way of survival, balance, and harmony for everything in the universe, but also way of balancing human mental health.

The Inner Canon of the Yellow Emperor, Basic Questions, Chapter Manifestation of Yin and Yang says, "Yin and yang are way of heaven and earth, great outlines of everything, parents of change, root and beginning of birth and destruction, and palace for Shen. Treatment of disease should be based on roots of yin and yang."

Chinese cultural essence for thousands of years can be refined as two words – yin and yang, and finally integrated into one word – Way. There is a way for every walk of life. A gentleman uses way to obtain wealth. Yin-Yang Tai Chi diagram has become a formula for correctly dealing with all problems and a trump for cultivating and enlightening Heart Shen. Its nature is following the trend and achieving moderation and peace. (See Figure 2-3)

Outer border line in the diagram represents that individual and external environment, including natural environment, social environment, study and work environment, family environment, relatives and friends, should be in a state of dynamic adjustment and moderate balance. Inner boundary line between yin and yang represents dynamic adjustment and peace in one's mind.

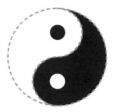

Figure 2-3   Dynamic balance of yin and yang in psychology

As a psychology counseling teacher in Shanghai University of Traditional Chinese Medicine, once I met a three-month freshman who often had conflicts with her Shanghai roommate but failed to rent an apartment outside the university due to family's financial condition. She came for help because of depressed emotion, which affects her study. During our conversation, I listened to her talk about how well her teachers and classmates treated her in high school in Harbin, and how well her parents and relatives treated her at home. In the end, I asked, "Where are you now?" She answered, "Shanghai!" I continued, "Then where is your heart?" She kept silent. I said, "You are in Shanghai, but your heart is still in Harbin. You have not adjusted yourself to new environment and campus culture in Shanghai. As Shanghai and Harbin are thousands of miles apart, their cultures are different. Conflicts between you and your roommate are caused by a clash of two regional cultures..." Finally, she said with enlightenment, "I will try to adjust myself. Then she left with a relaxed expression.

Different external stimuli, positive or negative, joyful or sorrowful, will always cause mood changes. Abiding extreme emotions will definitely cause change in corresponding viscera qi, leading to ups and downs in mood, lack of tranquility and purity, phlegm and stasis, turbid pathogens generating inside, dysfunction of viscera and bowels, and eventually developing into various mental diseases. *The Inner Canon of the Yellow Emperor, Basic Questions, Chapter Manifestation of Yin and Yang* says, "In human body, there are five viscera transforming five qi to generate joy, anger, anxiety, thought, and fear." TCM emphasizes that skilled doctors treat before sickness, which can also be applied in psychological counseling and treatment.

(2) BALANCE BETWEEN YIN AND YANG AND PEACE OF MIND

The Inner Canon of the Yellow Emperor, Volume Miraculous Pivot, Chapter Twenty-Five Yin-Yang Types classifies humans into twenty-five types of personality based on yin, yang, and five elements, and expounds on appearance, skin color, behavioral characteristics, and psychological traits of each type. Everyone is a unity of yin and yang. In different stages of life, or under different conditions of Shen, people will have different personalities. For instance, yin personalities include introversion, low profile, stingy, selfish, greedy, low self-esteem, laziness, indifference, and so on; yang personalities include extroversion, flamboyance, fanaticism, generosity, selflessness, dedication, self-confidence, diligence, enthusiasm, and so on. *The Inner Canon of the Yellow Emperor, Volume Miraculous Pivot, Chapter Needle Manipulation* says, "Those who have more yang qi tend to be joyful, and those who have more yin qi tend to be angry but can be relieved easily." It illustrates characteristics of those with partial personalities.

Chinese characters are main carriers of Chinese culture. Since creation by Cangjie, Chinese characters have undergone process of transforming pictograms into ideograms. Some Chinese characters even convey psychological knowledge. Taking character "心 (xin, heart)" as an example, from pictograms of oracle bone script, Chinese Bronze Inscriptions, and small seal script, to clerical script, regular script, and modern script, psychological meaning of character "heart" can be seen as follows: the vertical hook in the middle is shaped like a container, representing Heart's tolerance and openness; the left and right dots represent positive (yang) and negative (yin) experiences in the journey of Heart; and the middle point is to place moderate, right, and balanced things in Heart.

Characters composed of "心" include 思 (si, mind), 想 (xiang, idea), 意 (yi, thought), 念 (nian, missing), 怒 (nu, anger), 恐 (kong, fear), 悲 (bei, sorrow), 虑 (lv, contemplation), 志 (zhi, will), 愛 (ai, love). These characters are mostly related to spirit, consciousness, thought, and mental activity. If Heart does not make choices and regulations among various complicated experiences, it will be overburdened, resulting in psychological disorder and imbalance.

Characters composed of radical "忄 (heart)" are mostly related to emotions, moods, feelings and other activities, including 情 (qing, emotion), 惊 (jing, shock), 忧 (you, worry), 惧 (ju, fear), 恼(nao, annoyance), 愉 (yu, pleasure), 怅(chang, desolation), 恨 (hen, hatred), 忏 (chan, penance), 悔 (hui, reregt), 憾 (han, pity), 憎 (zeng, dislike), 悚 (song, horror), 怵 (chu, fear), 怔 (zheng, surprise), 悦 (yue, pleasure), 慌 (huang, panic), 愠 (yun, anger), 慎 (shen, prudence), 怡 (yi, cozy), 忆 (yi, memory), 愕 (e, startled), 愤 (fen, anger), 怯 (qie, fear), 惬 (qie, comfort), 慽 (qi, worry), 恤 (xu, compassion), 怅 (chang, melancholy), 惕 (ti, vigilance), 悸 (ji, fear), 懵 (meng, muddle), 懂 (dong, understand), 怜 (lian, pathy), 悯 (min, mercy), 怕 (pa, scare), 恫 (dong, intimidation).

Vertical line in the middle of "忄" represents that a person's overall emotion should be impartial, upright, neutral and peaceful. Left side represents yang and positive, while right side represents yin and negative. Left and right dots represent whether emotion is positive or negative, it should not stay on the middle line, nor on either side of the line. Any emotional manifestation of joy, anger, anxiety, thought, sorrow sadness, fear and fright should be immediate and transient. Any abiding, excessive, or extreme emotion will cause middle line leaning to left or right side. Long-term left or right partiality will lead to imbalance of five viscera qi, and thus disorder in five viscera Shen and even psychological imbalance and mental obscurity. Examples include Fan Jin passing Civil Exam, ecstasy leading to madness, fool's paradise, getting dizzy with success, etc.

2.6 Conclusion and Suggestion

(1) CONCLUSION

In summary, all psychological problems, including psychological disorders, psychopathology, personality bias, personality mutation, personality defects, personality alienation and even all spiritual, psychological and emotional diseases are more or less related to obscurity of Heart Shen. Brightness and obscurity of Heart Shen belongs to imbalance between yin and yang, a category of view on illness in TCM. Both healthy body and healthy mind use yin-yang balance as a benchmark.

As a grain of sand has a world, a person has his own world as well. Only the visitor himself knows whether his inner world is sunny or dark. One must take the initiative to open the window of his Heart and let sunshine in to fill his inner world with brightness. Whatever method is used, it is necessary to make visitor's Heart Shen back to brightness, that is, to restore normal cognition (brightness of self-knowledge). Only in this way can psychological diseases be cured completely.

Counselor should guide visitors to understand where their problems lie in and what they need to change, making them willing to change themselves from heart and gain willpower to self-cultivate and enlighten themselves, which can twice the effect with half the effort. This requires counselor to have a deep foundation for psychology. One should find interruption of emotions and confusion behind psychological phenomenon and purposefully guide visitors to solve psychological problems on their own. Psychological counseling that takes matter on its merits can only treat the tip and temporarily solve problem, or even increase visitors' psychological burden sometimes.

(2) SUGGESTION

As psychology practitioners and researchers, the first and foremost task is to make the public understand that mental health, mental normalcy, and personality soundness depend on their own conscious and purposeful self-cultivation, that a healthy and peaceful mind cannot be innate or naturally acquired, and that Heart Shen must be constantly cultivated and corrected to gradually become bright.

The Inner Canon of the Yellow Emperor, Basic Questions, Chapter Explanation for Acupuncture says, "Needling technique should be correct and straight down. After inserting the needle, look into patient's eyes to control his Heart Shen and thus make meridian qi flow smoothly." Relying on others for guidance and comfort to alleviate psychological problems is only makeshift. Cultivating and enlightening Heart Shen on one's own is way of treating the root.

LECTURE 3

The Stone of the Other Mountain

Localization of Clinical Psychology

LECTURER: HE YUMIN

Introduction to the speaker:

He Yumin, Professor, Doctoral Supervisor, Member of Chinese Medical Association and Former Chairman of Psychosomatic Medicine Branch, Vice-Chairman of Chinese Medical Philosophy Association, Advisor of Medical Humanities Committee of Chinese Medical Doctor Association, Editor-in-Chief of *Chinese Medical Encyclopedia Medical Psychology and Psychosomatic Medicine,* won China Lifetime Achievement Award of Psychosomatic Medicine, World Outstanding Chinese Achievement Award, Shanghai Labor Model and other awards. He also undertook a number of key projects of the Ministry of Science and Technology/National Social Science, and focused on refractory cancer treatment clinically.

Thank you for joining me in discussing the localization of clinical psychology, a big topic.

Psychological problems are not exactly the same as medical ones, and the former is more closely related to traditional culture. In fact, I often talked about this topic in the Congress before because the topic I did when I was a graduate student was psychological. In the 1990s, China established the Psychosomatic Medicine Branch of the Chinese Medical Association, and I was one of the founders. I have served as a vice-chairman for 14 years, two-term-chairmen for 6 years, and now I am a former chairman. Some people say that the 21st century is the century of the brain, the spirit and the mind. I think that is right. Why do we ask the question of localization of clinical psychology? Because in today's multicultural environment, we need to take into account all kinds of cultures.

Our ancestors has a thorough research on psychology, and there are a large number of systematic introductions in our ancient literature. Some are very interesting! This interesting is reflected in today's reference value. C.G. Jung, a well-known psychoanalyst, once made it clear that his thoughts were influenced by Taoism. Murphy, a famous American psychologist, also pointed out that the first home of world psychology is China. Therefore, it is problematic if we do not value traditional culture by ourselves.

3.1   The Origin of Research Psychology

I am personally interested in both psychological and medical disciplines. I think for the moment: according to strict scientific standards, psychology itself is not very mature; but the more immature the subject, the more opportunities. In addition, the subject is very active. At the annual meeting of the Psychosomatic Medicine Branch of the Chinese Medical Association in 2015, there were 700–800 participants. My topic is "*Clinician: Should Learn from Psychology Humbly.*" Clinicians give the impression that they are serious, stereotyped, disciplined and have lost their vitality. Of course, this is just my opinion. I am also a clinician, but I always feel that the clinician is stereotyped, not as humble, hard-working and progressive as a psychologist. I think clinicians (here, clinicians mean doctors who treat diseases) should learn from clinical psychologists well. This point of view has caused a great response, and I was invited to speak at their hospital on the spot. Researches on Humans psychological problems, spiritual (soul) problems, coupled with brain problems, are almost blank. Traditional Chinese medicine psychology is more immature than psychology, so we need to take a heart-strengthening agent.

3.2 Significance of psychosomatic research

I have been thinking the question that why should we do psychosomatic research for a long time, and the reasons are as below:

1) Many well-known scientists (including some Nobel Prize winners) who do brain research, such as Penfield who studies advanced brain and epilepsy, Sperry who does right/left brain function research, Eckles found that resistive synaptic potentials... These scientists have made great achievements in psychological (brain) research, but unfortunately, they still cannot explain many basic problems; therefore, they eventually converted to religion unexpectedly. In addition, I read an article: It is said that among the 1,000 scientists in the West, when they get old, 38% of them begin to believe in the existence of Spirit, and 39% believe in the existence of the post-mortem world (Nature, April 3, 1997). My understanding is that we could not explain so many fundamental problems, but rational scientists always need an explanation, a psychological trust, so they finally can only convert to religion. After a lifetime of research, many problems cannot be explained theoretically, so they can only rely on other understandings or even beliefs.

2) This field is very active but there are still too many blanks, which need us to study well.

3) There are many foreign psychological theories and heart-brain relationship hypotheses that we have introduced, most of which are not acclimatized. Although some are really good, but few really fit, because there are too many schools, opinions vary.

4) It is an urgent need for China to rise. I have always remembered a sentence: China can export socks, but not ideas, said a world-famous politician. I listened to this sentence at that time, not angry, but very confused: we have Confucius, Laozi and so on so many outstanding thinkers, how can we not export ideas? In our prosperous Tang and Song dynasties, what is the state of your Europe? Therefore, from this point of view, the export of TCM, although is very difficult, but the significance is prominent. Tu Youyou won the first Nobel Prize in Physiology or Medicine in China and made a great contribution. But its symbolic significance is far greater than the practical significance. Therefore, whether the modern significance of Chinese thought and Chinese tradition can be affirmed by the world depends on the Chinese people's contention.

In fact, I am very concerned about these. I have a national key social science project – *Research on Modern Transformation of the Core Value of Traditional Chinese*

Medicine Culture. Because transformation research needs to focus on many other related disciplines, such as politics, economics, law, philosophy, astronomy, geography and so on. In the field of politics, Chinese scholars' study of the World System, can you explain today's China with the Western set? No. In the field of philosophy, in the 1980s, we had a famous philosopher, named Li Zehou, very well-known! To what extent, the real overwhelming popularity of a new work causing shortage of printing paper! His books, many of them sold tens of millions, almost one person has one which is far more than today's superstars. A few years ago, at the age of 85, he wrote a book *The Philosophy of China Comes on Stage.* He originally talked about aesthetics, philosophy, etc. I consulted him a lot and communicated a lot. He asked me about health and I asked him about his philosophical proposition. Li said, This Chinese philosophy has come on the scene! Specifically, Western philosophy talks about ontology, starting with 'atom,' and continuing to talk about 'nihility,' discussing the meaning of existence (existentialism), and going on, it is impossible to talk about it! Later it may become more and more mysterious, more and more out of the `vernacular'. Back to reality, Chinese philosophy has come on stage, said Li. He emphasized that in the 1980s, when China talked about mind ontology and emotion ontology, when we considered philosophical issues, we could let the ancient Chinese express their opinions. Now there is no need to be so mysterious and ungrounded. The proposition of emotional ontology is to return to the reality of human life and daily life, which can also reveal many mysteries! China can provide the world with a source of ideas! And it's original!

In retrospect, the specific philosophical elucidation, we will not expand. At least 5000 years of ancient civilization, China has her deep culture. There are many good things we need to dig, refine, sublimate and think about! The world does not have only one plate (two Greek civilizations that the Western advocated), but has a variety of plates (culture and civilization). The world is essentially a big garden, flowers blossom together, the world will be full of spring and vibrant. Therefore, we should contribute to the field of medicine-related psychology. We are at best (worldwide) a listener who listens to what others say; then, like a tape recorder/microphone, disseminates the message and argues about some of their differences. We should strive to speak and need to say that they do not seem to have heard of it!... The foundation and basis can be the ideological wealth accumulated by history. But it is obviously not enough to talk about historical accumulation alone! At best, it's just speaking according to (the old ancestors), speaking along (the past) (which is called by a good name of inheritance); we still need to continue! (Promote the future). That is to say, on the basis of historical accumulation, we should make full use of it and combine with the progress of the times. In modern China, we need to be able to contribute a little intellectual wealth to the world, especially in the field of psychology. In addition to Tu Youyou's technical contribution artemisinin, I think psychology can also contribute a lot of things, including ideas, epistemology, theoretical interpretation, operational technology, etc.

This is the central idea of my speech, also the opening remarks!

In fact, before this, many scholars have done a lot of work (but not necessarily have conscious subjective consciousness, because in the past 150 years, Chinese self-esteem and self-confidence have been seriously damaged). For example, Pan Shu, the elder. Also, Professor Yan Guocai in Shanghai has made great achievements in his research on the history of ancient Chinese psychological thought. And Gao Juefu, the elder, has also done in-depth research. Including myself, I have also done some special research. In the 1990s, I wrote two books on this topic: one was *Traditional Chinese Tsychopathology* (1995). Unfortunately, the impact was not very great, because people didn't pay much attention to it at that time. The other one is *Pathology of Gender Differences in Traditional Chinese Medicine* (1997). It is found that the ancients have long recognized that there are great differences in psychological characteristics between men and women. Therefore, it is emphasized that many differences should be considered in clinical treatment between men and women. In the carding of psychological problems of traditional Chinese medicine, it is found that clinical psychological problems are often the premise of solving physiological problems. Again, the simplest words: my clinical job is to treat tumors, whether pancreatic cancer or liver cancer, you first have to face patients with pancreatic cancer or severe pain in the head of the pancreas and other problems, there is no fundamental solution! What should I do? First of all, it is necessary to solve psychological, emotional, cognitive and other issues, so that patients will have the hope of survival and may cooperate with active treatment. If the patient has already despaired, at this time, no matter how good the medicine is also invalid! The spirit and Qi transport medicine (Zhang Jingyue's words). You don't have a magic drug that can solve the cancer problem immediately. It's impossible! Therefore, we advocate to treat cancer from the heart! Self-summary: it is a relatively deep psychological background, which has helped me to achieve some achievements in the field of refractory tumor treatment. Perhaps, I am one of the domestic oncologists who actively develop psychology and have the deepest feelings about psychology. Generally speaking, for almost all refractory chronic diseases, if the doctor does not help the patient to establish a firm belief to live, and does not improve his bad mood and wrong cognition, it may be ineffective.

3.3   Localization of Psychology

As for the localization of psychology, I think it has three types (will be discussed later); localization also includes two major links, which need theoretical thinking, practice and specific operation (application).

3.3.1   The theoretical origin of Chinese psychology

The theoretical thought of Chinese psychology is very profound. It's just that we look at it with colored glasses (this pair of colored glasses is brought to us by western mainstream knowledge) to see if it fits in with the western set, and then we can select it according to the criteria. Moreover, the field of traditional Chinese medicine focused on the books of traditional Chinese medicine (focusing on those books that were abused), while the academic circle was limited to Confucius, Mencius, Laozhuang and Xunzi Guanzi. We did not calm down, broaden our horizons and explore them. In fact, many real and good things are not all in these classic works. There are a lot of psychological contents in the *Book of Songs*. Some scholars have done a good job in this respect. In Qian Zhixi's *View of Life Before Tang Dynasty and the Theme of Literary Life*, there are a lot of related contents when discussing the outlook on life. Therefore, in terms of theory, I will take some time to sort it out.

3.3.2   The application of psychology in China

Application can solve practical problems. Tu Youyou has won honor for the Chinese because artemisinin has saved millions of people in the world. Well, you have to admit that it works. Some theories like tumor are still unclear! However, with the help of psychology and psychosomatic medicine, many patients with advanced pancreatic cancer, liver cancer and brain tumor live well! You have to admit it.

3.3.3   Localization of Chinese psychology

There are at least three aspects of localization.

(1) Original.
   I think it's easier for us to recognize. It involves theory and application. Yang Desen, an old professor of Hu Nan Xiangya Medical College, I heard his

lecture in the 1980s. He is now old and should be over 90 years old. It is interesting that he created *Taoist Cognitive Therapy*. This is originality. Of course, theoretically, there are many original theories in Chinese traditions, which will be covered later.

(2) Improvement.

Just like another famous psychiatrist, Zhong Youbin, as you may know, he created the cognition and comprehension therapy with considerable insight. This is actually an improvement on the Western related therapy and integrates Chinese characteristics. Therefore, some people call him Freud of China.

(3) Grafting.

There are more grafts. This kind of grafting can be the grafting between the eastern and western psychology, or the grafting between different eastern disciplines (in fact, it is the mutual penetration of various disciplines). Mr. Xue Chongcheng's theory of five states of traditional Chinese medicine is to absorb (graft) the theory of five elements.

3.4   Research status of psychology in China

In any case, as a great country with a population of 1.3 billion and a history of 5000 years, we have little originality in the field of Psychology (psychosomatic medicine), and we are far from enough. There is a *Morita therapy* in Modern Japan, which left a mark in the history of related disciplines. Although some scholars think *Morita therapy* is not very practical and the improved version is not so practical, at least it is advocated by others. Science and technology only talk about originality! China has a lot of originality. But in the past hundred years, we have been poor and weak, and our sense of innovation has been exhausted. In fact, a closer look at China's export is quite a lot, such as relaxation therapy, more or less left China's birthmark. Biofeedback also has obvious traces of China. When I was a student, Professor Miller, the founder of biofeedback, had visited China, including the research institutes of our college. But these, at best, we only provide raw materials and blanks. After others borrow your ideas to improve, they innovate and become his things. For a long time, the Chinese did not consciously innovate. You can't even be conservative. Now when the world talks about yoga, it is known that it is India's business card. Prime Minister MoDi came to China and led Premier Li Keqiang to do yoga. But historically, Daoyin and tuna were very popular in 1000 BC. It originated from a kind of ceremony (which was the top priority at that time) and had various forms. To around A.D., its health care role has been not bad! And yoga in India's source, originally just a kind of religious ceremony! At least, we do not realize that we do not go deep into the excavation and promotion! There are many problems of this kind.

When I was a graduate student, one thing really stung me. At that time, the Chinese government began to award Natural Science Awards for the first time, and the only first prize was awarded to an Englishman, Joseph Needham. Needham deserves the prize. But the problem is that the prize is the research on the history of science and technology in China! As a big country, it boasts a profound cultural and historical tradition, and is especially good at culture, history and philosophy. However, its own history of scientific and technological development needs others (foreigners) to help you write (of course, we know that Needham invited some Chinese assistants to participate in the subsequent writing). Since then, I have focused on this field for decades, and bought too many works on the history of science and technology written by Chinese people in this field (including the newly published *General History of Science and Technology in China* with extremely luxurious binding and thick five volumes). Perhaps, the authors are well-known, but compared with Joseph Needham's earlier works, it can only be said that they are not in a heavyweight (the author has also concerned the criticism of the work). Why? Chinese people are not short of first-hand materials and other materials, as well as relevant wisdom, time and energy. However, what they lack is the cultural self-confidence, vision (horizon) and cognitive height of the whole nation's intellectuals, as well as the determination to go deep into themselves and do those researches seriously hard-working (perhaps pan Jixing's *History of Chinese Gunpowder* and *History of Chinese Papermaking* are exceptions). Chinese people have been beaten down for a period of time. They are self-enclosed (autistic) and lack of self-esteem and self-confidence.

This problem may be more serious in the field of traditional Chinese medicine. From time to time, there are so-called abolition of traditional Chinese medicine storm while psychology is no better which was often criticized in the 1950s and 1960s. Therefore, in these fields, we can make some original researches of China's own. Of course, in the field of clinical (medical) psychology, a lot can be done. The starting point of psychosomatic medicine in the world is not very high. The problems related to psychosomatic (brain) are complex and with too many blanks. Moreover, human beings are eager to fill in those blanks in these fields, so as to make people's body/mind/spirit fuller, so as to promote the improvement of human's overall psychosomatic quality. To sum up, I think our purpose is very clear! It is necessary and possible to improve clinical psychology in China. And it is likely to produce original results. These original achievements are often the fruits of localization.

3.5 The theory of localization of Clinical Psychology

It is very important to construct the theory of localization of clinical psychology, because the relevant knowledge can reach a new height of history and logic with the help of theory. The related theories of TCM (psychosomatic and psychological) are not only simple and dry as seven emotions, five minds, five zang-organs generate five minds and five emotions hurt five viscera. In fact, the relevant theoretical knowledge of traditional Chinese medicine (or Chinese traditional culture) is very rich.

3.5.1 Psychological structure

According to traditional Chinese medicine, mind and spirit have internal special structure, which is actually to understand people's psychological problems according to the holistic view with internal complete structure. As we all know: as far as mind and spirit (Psychology) is concerned, traditional Chinese medicine (TCM) is short for Shen, which has rich discussions. For example, in terms of the composition of *Divine Pivot-Benshen*, it said: what is the meaning of virtue and Qi generating essence, spirit, ethereal soul, corporeal soul, heart, mind, will, thought, wisdom and consideration? The two spirits fighting each other is called the spirit; those who follow the spirit are called ethereal soul; those who go in and out with the essence are called corporeal soul; therefore, those who allow things are called the heart; the heart that remembers is the meaning; the existence of the meaning is the will; the existence and change of the will is the thinking; the thinking and the distant admiration are the consideration; the thinking and dealing with the things are called the wisdom... That's enough.

The meaning is shown in Figure 3-1:

Psychic (divine)
- Instinctive activity — corporeal soul
- State of consciousness — ethereal soul
- Cognitive process
  - Memory — meaning
  - Thinking — Bunsen
  - Imagination — consideration
- Will process — will
- Intellectual activity — wisdom
- Emotional process: joy, anger, thinking, worry (sadness), fear (surprise)
- Sleep and dream

***Figure 3-1** Based on the discussion of* **Divine Pivot-Benshen**, *refer to the mental and psychological structure of traditional Chinese medicine (including emotion and sleep)*

Among them, spirit is the dominating and highly generalized, and is divided into Yin and Yang; Yin spirit is the corporeal soul and Yang spirit is the ethereal soul; a series of specific psychological activities and processes make them further evolved or controlled (we can also distinguish original spirit, conscious spirit and desire spirit, those details are as follow). Emotions also have a lot of branches. There are more than ten kinds of emotions. Sleep is also thought to be the result of the mind. In addition, there are essence, Qi and spirit theory, nature, emotions and desire theory, and free coursing of ministerial fire theory in TCM. A complete Gestalt structure of mental psychology in TCM is clearly visible. Moreover, according to our analysis, this Gestalt structure is far superior to the Gestalt School of German psychology.

On this basis, traditional Chinese medicine emphasizes that body and spirit are compatible and body and spirit are integrated. In today's words, they mean psychosomatic correlation and psychosomatic entanglement. Its performance is that the five viscera (especially the heart as the center), the five viscera are respectively linked to the five organs, five bodies, limbs fascia and other skeleton, and the meridians are widely belong to the collaterals, thus forming a Gestalt structure of the body. This structure is related to the above-mentioned heart-spirit structure, emphasizing the complex connection and interaction between different tissue structures (organs) and functional activities (mind and spirit). Although most of these understandings are conjectured and it is difficult to deconstruct the details by reductive methods, but they reflect more intertwined features between different things, and also enlighten people to pay attention to the fact that hyper-structural connections such as brain gut axis and lung blood production are explored.

In view of this, the author recently proposed the theory of heart-body entanglement (see *Medicine and Philosophy*, 2017. 7).

3.5.2 Psychosomatic relationship

If we say that the mind and body become a whole, there is still some consensus between China and the west, but there is a huge difference in the aspect of psychosomatic correlation: Western medicine almost does not involve this kind of connection. Even the most closely related major branches of psychosomatic medicine, behavioral medicine, and psychiatry are often vague, and each has its own niche. This is a big regret. In the traditional understanding of traditional Chinese medicine, the two are integrated into one like You have me, I have you and even you and I (spirit & mind body) are difficult to distinguish. The first paragraph of the first chapter of *The Inner Canon of the Yellow Emperor (On Ancient Original Qi)* sets the tone: ancient people, who knows, therefore, their body can integrate with their spirit, and the end of its life, they've already spent a hundred years. This can be analyzed from the following aspects:

(1) THE COMPLEXITY AND MULTIPLICITY OF CORRELATION

This is too complicated to be simply summarized according to traditional Chinese medicine, there is a general relationship between the body and the spirit, such as the heart, liver and spleen of the five viscera, which have the closest relationship with spirit, blood nourishing spirit, emotion disordering Qi mechanism, and so on. There are also specific corresponding relations, such as the five viscera generating five minds (the liver has the mind of anger), the five minds damage the five viscera (anger hurts liver), Five viscera in charge of different organs (the lung opens the orifices in the nose, the sense of smell), and so on. Moreover, this kind of correlation involves almost all the physical organs and mental and psychological aspects, which will not be repeated here because of its complexity.

(2) THE RELATIONSHIP BETWEEN FORM AND SPIRIT

If we do not explore the origin of the mind body and the inner deep relationship, we can only discuss the phenomenon of body-spirit/mind-body interaction in a plane way, which is impossible. In terms of the origin of the mind and body, people have different opinions. The author has summarized more than ten hypotheses at home and abroad (see *Clinical Research of Traditional Chinese Medicine Psychology* for details). I have to think that the theory of distinguishing heaven from nature which originated in the Jin Dynasty (liuhejian) and matured in the Ming and Qing Dynasties is quite insightful. For example, Qi Shi, a famous doctor in the early Qing Dynasty, said: if the body theory is based on the innate generation, then the essence will generate Qi and Qi will generate the spirit; if the theory is based on the domination of the acquired usage, then the spirit will serve Qi and Qi will serve the essence. In terms of genealogy, the essence (including the brain and other organs and tissues) produces Qi (functional activity), and Qi (functional activity) is associated with spirit (Mental Psychology); however, once the spirit is produced, it can control the function (spirit controls Qi) and further control the body viscera (Qi controls essence). It not only affirms the primacy of matter in genealogy, but also points out its decisive significance after its emergence. It is much more incisive than the vulgar philosophical cliche of spirit changing material and material changing spirit. Comparative analysis shows that this view is the same as that of W.R. Sperry, who won the Nobel Prize in physiology or medicine for schizencephalon research in

1980s. Sperry's conclusion is that the new feature of consciousness as a whole activity at all levels in the subcortical region is not the sum of simple neuro physical chemical events, but once it emerges, it has a decisive effect on the lower layers. It is not too much to say that this view of Qi Shi is the origin of Si's theory.

(3) The heart integrates the functions of the mind (see Figure 3-2)

Plain Questions Ling Lan mysteries emphasizes that the heart is the official of the monarch, and the mind come out. *Miraculous Pivot Evil on the Opponents' Field* says that the heart is the master of the five viscera and six bowels, and the place of the spirit. In modern words, heart integrates the two functions of form and spirit, making it more orderly and coordinated. If we further consider the difference between the heart of flesh and blood and the heart of mind; the latter refers to the brain, the problem will be clearer.

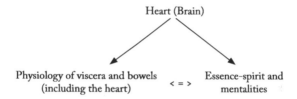

Figure 3-2   Heart integrates the function of body and spirit

(4) Phenomenological study of mind body conjugation

The author pays special attention to the psychosomatic problems. In the past 30 years, several large sample epidemiological studies have been carried out to reveal the complex relationship between mind and body.

1) Preliminary conclusion of constitution temperament research

In the 1980s and 1990s, the author was addicted to the study of the relationship between constitution and temperament. Instead of the normal (referring to ancient medical books and subjective identification items), the author followed the principle of scientific methodology and took the lead in introducing mathematical methods such as fuzzy clustering and neural network. He emphasized that starting from facts and based on sufficient objective data, the author borrowed several revised CCQ and DPQ Using the probability and condition introduction formula, the correlation coefficient was calculated and fuzzy clustering was carried out. According to the conclusion of fuzzy clustering and referring to the experience of medical theory and experts, the final result was determined. For example, in terms of constitution, three main types and several subtypes can be clearly found: strong type; weak type; maladjusted type. Among them, there are a series of subtypes under each main type, and the most subtypes of maladjustment type are similar to the clinical description of traditional Chinese medicine.

With the same method (only different questionnaires), the temperament/personality factors related to the disease can be clearly clustered. The common ones are: introversion; sense of time urgency (urgency/slowness); hostility and competition (they are highly positively correlated, and there is no need to distinguish them by force); depression; tolerance; emotional instability; and anxiety.

Moreover, there is an interesting correlation between different temperament/personality: for example, extroversion and acuteness, extroversion and hostile competition, there is a significant positive correlation between two. People with depression is more likely to be introverted; people with a quick and slow temperament have nothing to do with depression; People with expression are often full of hostility. The most important significance of cluster study is to reveal the close relationship between constitution and temperament/personality. *Psychosomatic Medicine* (2000) disclosed some conclusions of relevant studies: for example, extroversion and strong constitution showed a very significant positive correlation, but it was significantly negatively correlated with all the asthenia, weakness and biased maladjustment. It is suggested that physical strength is the physiological basis of extroversion; the weakening and deterioration of physique (maladjustment and bias) will weaken people's personality characteristics such as liveliness, enthusiasm, activeness and active communication.

Acute child has certain correlation with all physical types. But the highest positive correlation value was with robustness. As it may be said, strong physique people show more sense of time urgency.

Insufficiency of essence and blood was also positively correlated with sense of time urgency. It seems that the patients with deficiency of essence and blood mainly belong to the deficiency of Yin in liver and kidney, which is easy to be irritable, which can be explained by the theory of traditional Chinese medicine.

Hostility and competition are only highly positively correlated with strong physique, indicating that physical state is the capital of mental and psychological activities. Only those who are physically strong and energetic will be ambitious, have a strong sense of competition, and remain alert to many surrounding phenomena.

Depression is highly positively correlated with all types of weakness, disorder and other pathological constitutions, but negatively correlated with strength alone. It suggests that depression is closely related to physical condition. Strong people are less depressed, weak and disordered people are more depressed.

Tolerance is negatively correlated with weakness, heat, dampness, stasis, etc. It is also negatively correlated with cold and deficiency of essence and blood. There is no such relationship with strength alone. It may be explained that people with disordered and weak constitution are not very good at giving in. Tolerance also needs to be based on a certain physical basis.

Emotional instability was positively correlated with anxiety, all disorders and weaknesses, but negatively correlated with the strong. It suggests that when the constitution is weak or disordered, emotional instability and anxiety are very easy to occur, especially in the weak. On the contrary, people with strong physique seldom suffer from emotional instability and anxiety.

This is the conclusion drawn in the 1980s and 1990s in scientific research projects supported by Shanghai Municipal Education Commission. It can be seen that the conclusion of clustering is quite enlightening: physique is closely related to temperament/personality; generally, physical status (physique) is the basis; good physique will have a stable and good temperament/personality/mood and so on.

2) Conclusions from sub-health studies

In 2006, in the Key Supported Project of the 11th Five-Year Plan of the Ministry of Science and Technology, *Research on Measurement and Diagnostic Criteria of Subhealth*, we integrated the analysis of social-psychological-physical and other elements: The common state or symptoms in the physical field are divided into nine categories: fatigue, digestion, sleep, dysfunction, immunity, allergy, aging, pain and constipation; the common tendencies in the psychological field are briefly divided into two categories: depression and anxiety; the social field is divided into four major aspects: social support, social pressure, social adaptation, self-confidence and satisfaction ("properties" is deleted due to reliability problems); A survey of over 15,000 sub-healthy people, using structural equation model and other analysis and evaluation, finally showed that: there is a clear "conjugation phenomenon" between psychological and physical – the path coefficient of psychological factors affecting the physical field is 0.79, very high; the influence of physical on the psychological is 0.14, much weaker. However, the influence of social factors on physical physiology is often not a direct effect, which needs to be mediated by psychological factors, and then indirectly acts on the body. The indirect effect of social factors on the body is the product of two path coefficients ($0.68 \times 0.79 = 0.54$); the effect is also relatively strong and obvious.

Simply put, with the help of popular methods and structural equation models, it is found that there is a close interaction between the mind and the body; and the direction and strength of its role can be clearly shown by mathematical means (see Figure 3-3).

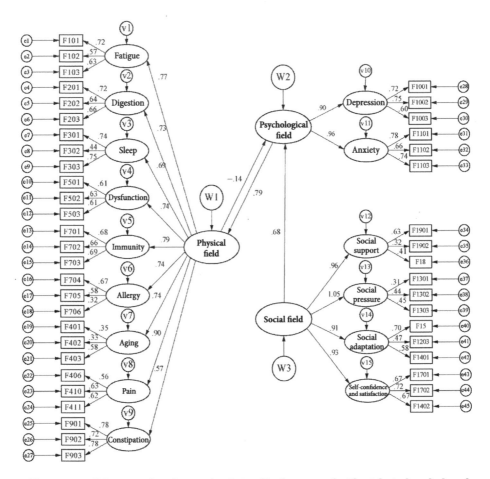

Figure 3-3   Discovery of psychosomatic relationships by means of epidemiological methods and structural equation models

It is well known that the shelf on the back of a cow is called a yoke, which is in the form of a "⌒". If one side of the yoke fails, it must affect the other side. This is called conjugation. Conjugation is commonly used in academic circles to refer to the related things that have a certain close relationship and interact with each other at all times. Based on this, we propose the phenomenon of mind-body conjugation.

3.5.3 Polarity characteristics of mind-body relationship

The existence of the phenomenon of "mind-body conjugation" is recognized by all contacting clinicians. In depth, there is an interactive relationship between these moments, presenting obvious "polarity" characteristics. The so-called "polarity" refers to the use of chemical terms, also known as "chirality" (left-handed/right-handed), referring to such mind-body interaction relations because of their different directions of action, the results are very different (like the two ends of a magnet or suction or mutual exclusion of the "polarity"); also like some compounds, although the molecular formula is the same, but the chirality is different, presenting different left-handed, but can be good drugs or highly toxic, respectively). Psychosomatic interaction can be a mutual benign promotion; it can also be an ever-increasing negative cycle – there are classical terms in traditional Chinese medicine to describe this negative interaction: "pathogenic due to depression," "depression due to illness."

The author deeply feels the distinct consequences of this "polar" interaction in the clinical oncology: too many successful convalescents, medical measures are one of the guarantees of their success, and the gradual formation of positive and benign mind-body interaction is the intrinsic mechanism to ensure their better recovery, which can be called "mind-body left-turn"! And the same too many recovery losers are entangled in a certain link of the body and mind and self-negative circulation – "illness" and "depression" between the constantly present inferior amplification effect (similar to the "mind-body right-handed"), and ultimately sink, it is gripping!

For example, not only cancer, but also all areas of medical concern – from health/sub-health to morbidity, as well as common diseases with close mind-body interaction (coronary heart disease, hypertension, diabetes, peptic ulcer, etc.) should follow the value of striving to promote the "mind-body left-turn" of the service object; and methodologically it is advisable to adopt a "bringing doctrine" attitude and choose various mature therapies/means. Include the creation of new methods/measures as long as the results are conducive to forming a positive "mind-body left-handed" relationship. Including sub-health areas. Several years ago, more than 15,000 subjects were investigated in the study of "Preventive treatment and sub-health," a major national scientific research project. Further analysis revealed that there were "leverage factors" in the transition from health to sub-health and from sub-health to morbidity; among the "leverage factors," the highest risk factor was "individual satisfaction with self." This is a sociological concept. But if we learn to adjust our understanding, optimize our values, and learn to be happier, we may avoid many diseases. The following dangerous "leverage factors" are "persistent fatigue" and "insomnia," etc., which are also common and potential threat factors that need to be corrected.

Emphasizing the "polarity" effect of mind-body relationship, its significance lies in prompting and emphasizing: to cure diseases and maintain health, we should cut into the two links of mind-body. This is what TCM calls "preventive treatment" and "the best work is to guard peoples mind." Some old TCM doctors may first play a role of psychological hint when treating a patient; patients believe in them, psychological lead into a virtuous circle. Are there any bad effects of psychological hint? No.

Based on the above understanding of TCM, we redefine psychosomatic medicine as "recognizing and focusing on psychosomatic interaction (including health, disease and the whole life process), and trying to promote the formation of positive psychosomatic interaction by means of various methods, in order to keep healthy, prevent disease or promote recovery, or promote the improvement of quality of life." Although this is only a functional and objective definition, because it integrates the local wisdom of TCM psychology, its guidance in preventing and treating diseases is more prominent. If we communicate around the world, we may have more Chinese characteristics.

3.5.4 Rational Understanding of "Instinct" in Traditional Chinese Medicine

Instinct is an important proposition in psychology. Western scholars, whether Freud's Dynamics School, Maslow's humanism, or Marcuse's theory of "eroticism," all attach importance to the issue of human instinct, and believe that "instinct" is the internal driving force of life activities. Instinct refers to a natural tendency, which is not only due to the animal attributes of human beings, but also a kind of psychological activities and behavioral responses; it is also inextricably linked to the social attributes of human beings; and is subject to the social environment and civilized norms of individual survival. Conflicts between instinct and reason, desire and reality, motivation and behavior constitute the deep roots of a variety of psychosomatic disorders, psychosomatic disorders and clinical psychological problems. Therefore, it is impossible to bypass the problem of "instinct" when we know all kinds of human activities.

Freud believed that instinct belonged mainly to the subconscious category. Although there is no clear concept of subconsciousness in traditional Chinese culture, scholars in Song Dynasty put forward similar concepts of "The spirit is dormant in the brain. "and" The spirit is contained in the inner organs "in their exploration of dreams, and some connotations such as "seal," "off-line," "dejavu" and "hermit" have appeared, which are far beyond the "subconsciousness." At the same time, inspired by Cheng Zhu's Confucian school of idealist philosophy of the Song and Ming dynasties, the medical profession established the instinct theory with "liver governing free flow of qi" as the main body. Relevant concepts such as human desire, desire spirit, ministerial fire, free flow, forming a series of specific concepts such as articulation, relaxation, rising, ministerial fire, sovereigned fire, Tao mind, human mind, hiding and storing, depression and stagnation and so on; and constructed a unique instinct theory in China.

(1) "Ministerial fire" – the natural instinct of a man who cannot be restrained

Early physicians did not pay attention to the term "free flow" nor regarded it as a major physiological and pathological concept. However, in the Southern Song Dynasty, the duality of human instinct and its relationship with health and disease were profoundly elaborated by Confucian doctors and Zhu Danxi, which had a solid foundation of Neo-Confucian. He put forward the theory of human desire, discussed the instinctive problems such as desire, pointed out that "human desire is endless," "The gentleness was in his body, the voice was in his ears, the color was in his eyes, and the fragrance was in his nose. Who was an iron man, and his heart was unmoved"? These desires, the impulses related to food, color, etc., are human instincts. As early as the pre-Qin period, *Mencius* recorded "food, color and properties." This issue is also discussed in *Xunzi Properties Evil*. Zhu Danxi regards it as a kind of internal impulse related to the nature of human nature. It is believed that it is on this "movement" that talent can survive and be full of vitality, and that the germline also depends on it to continue ("Man has this life because he always moves"). He borrowed the "Ministerial fire" from *The Inner Canon of the Yellow Emperor* to characterize this impulse. Emphasis: "People can't live without this fire (Ministerial fire)."

(2) From "Ministerial fire" to "free flow," dual significance to health

According to Zhu Danxi, as an instinct originating from the natural nature of human animals, Ministerial fire (or "lust impulse") has obvious duality: on the one hand, it is the intrinsic motive force for the continuation of the individual germline of life; on the other hand, this instinctive desire, often prone to delusions, frequently occurs, "Ministerial fire is prone to, Delusions are over. "Too frequent and strong desire impulse can damage the shape of life, so it is said: "Ministerial fire, the thieves of vitality." At the same time, Zhu Danxi connected the Ministerial fire with the liver (for the reason, they all started from the understanding of "the liver ascends actively, exhilarates, and represses evil." Various desires and impulses also have the characteristics of initiative, from inside to outside, so they are connected with each other). He pointed out that "Yin of liver and kidney, all have Ministerial fire." In the same article, Zhu Danxi bundled the "liver," "Ministerial fire" and "free flow" together and proposed that "the main reservoir, the kidney; the Department of free flow, the liver as well. Both viscera have fire, which is attached to the heart. The heart, the sovereign fire, is easily moved by things. The hearts and the ministerial fire affect with each other. When they move, the essence goes and the ministerial fire goes up. Although they do not meet, they also secretly free flow. This passage establishes the well-known theory of liver governing free flow of qi and forms the "instinctive theory" of China. Among them, the so-called "it belongs to the heart" and "the heart" or "the movement of heart" actually refer to the concept of "consciousness of mind" which will be discussed in the next section. Therefore, in Zhu Zi's theory, there are such concepts as origin of spirit, consciousness spirit and desire spirit. "Ministerial fire" means "desire spirit" and "Ministerial fire" means "free flow"; it is controlled by the understanding and thinking of "heart," that is, "consciousness Spirit."

(3) ESSENTIAL INTENTION OF FREE FLOW: HUMAN INSTINCTIVE DESIRE AND IMPULSE

Why use the word "free flow"? Literally, "Shu" means to dredge, while "Xie" means to let off. They both are the process from the inside to the outside, similar to the various desires and pursuits in human social life that are initiated from the heart and directed to the outside. After careful study of Zhu's said above: liver governing free flow of qi, the kidney governing the seal of qi, both of them are related to sexual function, Zhu believed that both "have ministerial fire"; Ministerial fire (desire spirit) is often caused by the heart induced by external things (here, "for things to feel but easily moved" heart, that is to say, "consciousness of the spirit" sprouting later), that is to say, common through the sense of Spirit. This impulse originally hides in the liver and kidney of the lower energizer... But they always point out. This is somewhat similar to Freud's. However, although the free flow here has been linked to the desire and impulse of the liver and instinct, it still has some distance from the meaning of the modern custom, it can only simply refer to the semen discharge in sexual activities, at best, is an external manifestation of the intrinsic instinct (Ministerial fire), or its visible results.

We will analyze later generations' understanding of this theory and its practical implications:

The popular textbooks of basic theory of traditional Chinese medicine often regard "liver governing free flow of qi" as having the following functions:

1) Promote the transportation of the spleen and stomach, ensure good appetite and normal digestive function;

2) Promote the normal secretion and excretion of bile, which is helpful to the transportation of the spleen and stomach;

3) Maintain the normal sexual function of men and women, ejaculation of men, menstruation and ovulation of women, etc.;

4) Participate in the operation process of regulating blood and body fluid in the body, so as to make them go in an orderly way; and

5) Maintain the mental and emotional state of people, Stability, harmony and smoothness; TCM theory calls it "smooth mood";

6) smooth qi movement.

And what TCM calls "Qi movement" is very similar to the autonomic nervous system. Therefore, the smooth regulation of Qi movement can make the whole-body visceral function coordinated, and the physiological processes smooth, neither weak nor hyperactive.

In a word, if livers free flow of qi is normal, the individual can be harmonious and stable in many aspects of physiology and psychology. Otherwise, they often fall into the pathological state of psychosomatic abnormalities. In view of this, through layers of veils, combined with the understanding of human nature by ancient sages and the related progress of psychosomatic medicine, it can be said that "free flow" is the euphemism used by ancient physicians to refer to human instinctual desire and impulse; "liver governing free flow of qi" is that "liver" is in charge of such desire impulses.

3.5.5 Traditional Chinese Medicine's Understanding of Deep Psychology

Traditional Chinese medicine believes that "Spirit" itself is very intricate and has a multi-level relationship. After the Ming Dynasty, TCM doctors were inspired by traditional culture, deepened the exploration of deep mental problems, and put forward enlightening insights. Today, it's just a brief introduction.

(1) Original spirit, desire spirit and consciousness spirit theory

After Song and Ming Dynasty, some doctors, influenced by Jin and Yuan Dynasty's exploration of the original style of life, began to explore the complex deep psychological problems from the perspective of Original spirit, desire spirit and consciousness spirit. In the meantime, a lot of knowledge is complementary to the above instinct theory.

1) Original spirit: Dominant Life – Similar to Central Regulation

Zhang Jingyue said, "Spirit has the original spirit, Qi has the original spirit. "Original spirit sees that Yuan Qi generates, and Yuan Qi generates Yuan Jing *Classic of Classics*. In Zhang's eyes, Original spirit seemed to be the leader. This knowledge is actually based on the health care family and Taoist.

Zhang Boduan of the Northern Song Dynasty said in the *Tips for Refining Dance in Jinbao*: "The spirit has an original spirit and a desire spirit. Original spirit is a bit of spiritual light since birth; the desire spirit is also the nature of gas endowment (the nature of gas endowment can be understood as the nature of the source animal)." Later, Yang Dao-sheng said in True Interpretation: "Or asking the Spirit of origin and thinking about Spirit is one and two. Say: Heart, properties, Spirit, too. With its endowment in the sky a little wise, so called the Spirit of Spirit. Later, it was moved by emotion, and this original spirit was not in emotion, and became the Spirit of thought (i.e., 'onsciousness spirit')."

In a word, Original spirit was originally a Taoist concept. Taoists believe that it comes from the innate, "the innate is the original Spirit as well" which is the dominant of life, "the original spirit, that is, the dominant in my true heart also" (Huang Yuanji: *Yueyutang Records*). It attaches itself to the skeleton for life, and to the flesh for death. Therefore, Taoists attach special importance to original spirit and advocate that health preservation and cultivation should be "used by Original spirit." For example, Zhao Taiding of Ming Dynasty emphasized in *Pulse Observation*: "If a person can hold the Spirit of origin and live in this palace, then the true Qi rises and the true truth is self-determined. The so-called "one knows and one knows and one knows and one knows and one knows and one knows all together." "He also advocated that "daily effort should be mainly focused on the Spirit of origin." What is the original spirit? It is called the original spirit because it does not originate from the inner thoughts, but is inconceivable from the outer thoughts and is independent of itself. "Among them, "the inner thoughts do not sprout" can be understood as the desire spirit has not sprouted; "the outside thoughts do not sprout" that is, the conscious spirit rests; at this time, the role of the dominant life is the original spirit.

In view of the great significance of original spirit, consciousness and desire spirit in traditional mental thoughts, it is necessary to make some explanations with the help of modern knowledge. In summary, the "Original spirit" seems to have several characteristics: (1) It is innate, people born with it, there is life; the original spirit leaves, life immediately terminates; (2) It is not governed by consciousness and so on, can play a role autonomously; and the conscious (consciousness and so on) depends on it to produce, although after the generation cannot dominate the original spirit, but can interfere with the original spirit, affect its control of life; (3) original spirit in the brain, not in the heart. In Li Shenzhen's *Compendium of Metromedia*, there is a saying: "Brain is the house of Original spirit." Zhao Taiding said in *Pulse Observation*: "Brain is the palace where Shang dan Tinoridine spirit resides." Zhang Xicheng also said: "The human Spirit is in the brain, and the conscious spirit is in the heart. The heart and brain are interlinked, and their spirits are self-conscious and awake" (*Shenxi Lu in The Heart of Medicine*); and (4) the spirits of origin play a role all the time and are the masters of life activities, and their soundness is "true Qi rises spontaneously, truth is self-determined" and "self-determination." Qigong meditation methods such as tranquility and pranayama have the effect of promoting the Spirit of origin to regulate life better (eliminating the interference of desire spirit and consciousness spirit on the Spirit of origin when tranquilizing, so they have this effect). Based on the above characteristics, combined with the modern understanding of the structural characteristics of the brain, it seems reasonable to conclude that the "original spirit" was a rough grasp of the central functions of life at all levels in the regulation of visceral activity under the cerebral cortex by ancient physicians, which included the lower evolutionary level of the medial cortex (mainly the limbic system) and the lower level of the hypothalamus, brainstem and other structures in which part of the regulatory role was played. Internal. It is essentially autonomous/ autonomous, usually less controlled by the idea ("autonomy alone, so-called original spirit"), similar to the autonomic nervous system center; but well-trained people can make some degree of self-feedback regulation by means of the idea under certain conditions. Just as well-trained Qigong masters or practitioners can often regulate certain organ functions to a certain extent.

It is clear that such regulatory functions as the origin spirit do exist, and they are born with the key to maintaining life.

2) Consciousness spirit – Supervisor Conscious Thinking

"Awareness of Spirit" is the original Buddhist concept, which refers to the spiritual entity that bears the causal reward in the theory of reincarnation. Taoists borrow to express mental activities such as thinking and consciousness, so they are sometimes called "thinking Spirit." It is a kind of activity based on the original spirit, which can interfere with the original spirit after it is produced ("the original spirit is not in the emotion"). Therefore, the Taoist family maintains their health by rejecting "conscious Spirit," "refining the Taoist Tao with the Spirit of origin" and "using the Spirit of origin with the Spirit of origin without thinking about the Spirit of origin." Consciousness can be approximated as the high-level psycho-psychological activities such as perception, thinking and consciousness generated by the neuro-electrochemical activities in the cerebral cortex, which are based on the activities of the lower level of the subcortical brain (i.e., the "spirits") and are generated after the stimulation of the external situation. Since it often interferes with the lower level of central regulatory functions in the subcortex, so as to affect the autonomous regulatory functions of these centers (i.e., the "original spirits"), and is not conducive to the regular physiological activities of the zang-fu organs, the health-care and Taoists advocate denouncing the "mind-seeking" and using the "original spirits."

3) Desire spirit – Instinct Desire Impulse

The Taoist saying of "desire spirit" includes all kinds of intrinsic desire impulses, which have the same meaning as the aforementioned "free flow" and "ministerial fire." Its movements also often interfere with the original spirit (original qi). Therefore, physicians and Taoists in the past dynasties often warned of "clearing the mind from desires," "idleness from desires," "tranquility and nihility" to "refresh the mind" and "whole spirit." Its purpose is to self-control the desire spirit and control it as much as possible so as to prevent its harassment of the original spirit and avoid the depletion of the original spirit.

4) There is an intricate hierarchical relationship between mind and mind.

Through the deduction of traditional Chinese medicine and Chinese traditional culture, we can find that behind the above theoretical hypothesis, there are still profound connotations, revealing the different associations between the mind and mind:

1) Low-level "desire spirit" – from "body" to "heart." As mentioned earlier, Chinese ancestors developed the theory of desire spirit, consciousness spirit and original spirit. The so-called "desire spirit" can be regarded as a kind of desire impulses and corresponding behaviors that generally refer to human beings originating from their individual biological instincts. The main manifestations are food, color (properties) and the tendency to benefit and avoid harm. It is closely related to the survival of individuals and the reproduction of populations. Essentially, such behavior is purely physical and physiological in animals, and is a purely physiological behavioral response under the control of the nervous system. But the situation is slightly different in humans. Although sometimes such behavioral responses can occur or proceed in an unconscious state, in most cases, individuals are clearly aware of the germination of such impulses and often make some kind of regulation with the aid of consciousness, at the same time, they are often accompanied by certain emotional experiences. That is to say, it also has some subordinate mental and psychological characteristics in humans, so ancient Chinese sages called it "desire spirit."

In this level of mind-body relationship, physical factors often play a causal/ decisive role. In terms of biological studies, the neuroregulatory centers that control such behavioral responses are located in relatively ancient structures (paleocortex, paleocortex, also known as limbic forebrain) from a biological evolutionary point of view. It can be said that the instinctive desire impulse is controlled by these system functions of the brain. However, traditional theory also holds that "consciousness spirit" can induce (or inhibit) desire spirit. From the biological mechanism, this is the result that the cortical neuro-electrochemical reactions accompanied by the activities of perception and consciousness in the cerebral cortex have a regulatory effect on the lower cortical centers. Essentially, this relationship is a descending effect of the body (cortical electrochemical reaction) on the body (limbic system function). In addition, some physicians, Buddhists and Taoists also emphasize that "desire spirit" can upstream interfere with the "original spirits" and affect the "consciousness spirit"; it can not only interfere with the regulation process of the life center ("the thieves of fire-generating qi"), but also affect the physiological activities of the viscera and other organs; it can also "disturb the consciousness spirit," affecting the perception, thinking and consciousness of the cortex, which is a common phenomenon. But in terms of primary and secondary, this ascending disturbance seems to be secondary to and weaker than the domination and manipulation of lust by the conscious spirit.

2) Original spirit from body to body. "Original spirit" has been interpreted before, which can be approximated as an understanding of the central function of life in regulating visceral activities under the cerebral cortex by ancient sages. In terms of structure, it is in close proximity to lust, including the regulation of parts of the medial cortex (mainly the limbic system) at lower evolutionary levels, the brainstem at lower levels, and the hypothalamus. These sites regulate visceral function mainly through autonomic nervous system and endocrine. This function is innate, and the limbic system is its regulatory center. Therefore, it can be said that "Original spirit" is mainly a neuro-electrochemical activity, belonging to the category of "body." But this function is also affected by the cerebral cortex, that is, the traditional theory called "conscious spirit" can interfere with or even control the "spirit." Because the parts are similar, some are different functions of the same structure, so the "desire spirit" and "original spirit" often affect each other.

3) Psychosomatic relationship of "conscious spirit": Chinese theory of "emergence." Consciousness of mind seems to be a kind of high-level psycho-psychological activities such as perception, thinking and consciousness

generated by neuro-electrochemical activities in the cerebral cortex. They are based on the activities of the lower level of the brain under the cortex (i.e., the "spirits") and are generated after the stimulation of the external situation. Through the modern research of brain science, it is gradually recognized that this kind of mental and psychological phenomena is manifested by the neural activity of the cerebral cortex and even the whole brain as a mechanism[1]." The subcortical structure plays a role in uploading and transmitting neurological information and maintaining the state of cortical arousal. These are of fundamental significance for the generation of thinking, consciousness, etc. Studies have confirmed that the cortex and neuro-electrochemical activities in the posterior part of the cerebral hemisphere are the final integration sites that directly cause psychological phenomena such as perception and consciousness. The neurochemical activities in other parts of the cerebral cortex can produce the above psychological phenomena only by causing the neuro-electrochemical activities in this part of the cerebral cortex. These sites are considered the highest level of human brain evolution.

The mind-body relationship at the level of "consciousness spirit" is the highest level and the most intricate and confusing. Perception, thinking, consciousness and so on are the characteristics of the cerebral cortex (the key is the posterior cortex) and the whole brain on the basis of neuro-electrochemical activity, so the body (brain, etc.) is the biological mechanism of the heart (perception and consciousness, etc.), and the heart "depends on the body" and "emergence"; but once the sense and consciousness are generated, they play a certain role in the neuro-electrochemical process of the brain. The regulatory role of properties. It not only regulates emotional responses and controls visceral activities through the circuits of the neocortex, limbic forebrain, anterior thalamic nucleus and hypothalamus, but also makes timely, precise and effective innervation of muscles and motor organs through the corresponding motor areas, pyramidal system, extrapyramidal system and motor nerves of the cerebral cortex. In these processes, the perception and consciousness derived from "conscious spirit" play a causal regulatory role on the somatic response process including cortex. It is based on the genius intuition of this relationship that TCM emphasizes the "spirit can

1. "Emergence" is a commonly used term in the interpretation of mind-body relationship by western scholars recently, which means: Psychological activity is the manifestation of a concentrated and sudden transition based on the overall function of the brain. It cannot be simply reduced to some neurological processes, and emphasizes that psychosocial activity is corresponding to the whole brain function rather than to a certain part.

hold shape" from a functional point of view. Moreover, the word "hold" here has the meaning of driving and controlling, which is far more pleasant and refined than the "spiritual reaction to material" commonly used in dialectical materialism. As far as this layer of mind-body relationship is concerned, 'body' (cerebral cortex and its activities) is the basis, and 'heart' (thinking, consciousness, i.e., 'consciousness') is the characteristic or result of 'body emergence'. But once the "mind" (consciousness of mind) emerges, it has a dominant and regulatory effect on the "body" and the lower level of the heart and body. The latter is precisely the factual basis on which "conscious spirit" influences "original spirits" and "conscious spirit" induces or inhibits "desirous spirit" and another related knowledge.

These localized understandings, after a little improvement, can not only serve as an important ideological source for our innovation in relevant fields, but also be beneficial to the acceptance of the civilian people after popular expression, thereby improving the self-awareness and level of mental and physical health, but also are valuable resources for us to make original in-depth research and put forward new theories.

3.5.6 Localization of Psychopathology

The aforementioned theoretical problems are mainly confined to the clinical psychological (physiological) part, in fact, TCM involves more pathology and clinical. First is the understanding of the psychological causes. Here, I do not want to repeat the well-known theory of pathogenicity of seven emotions and so on, but to make some new explanations on the less discussed/or changed perspective of people:

(1) DEPRESSION AS THE SOURCE OF ALL DISEASES – THE CORE OF PSYCHOLOGICAL CAUSES

Zhu Danxi has a well-known statement: "Qi and blood wash together, all diseases do not occur; when there is depression, all diseases occur. The diseases of the deceased are mostly due to depression." Many disciples of Zhu's family and private Shu, such as Wang Ru, Yi Silan, a famous doctor in the Yuan Dynasty, have repeatedly emphasized that "depression is the source of all diseases," "all diseases are born with depression." They have never tired of demonstrating the universality and harmfulness of depression syndrome. And the depression syndrome is also called "liver depression," "liver Qi depression," "liver depression and Qi stagnation." In fact, it reveals the etiology and pathological mechanism of psychosomatic (physical and mental) diseases, the core of that liver fails to govern free flow of qi. Therefore, it is worthwhile to make some analysis and modern elaboration in combination with clinical practice.

1) The universality of depression

"Depression is the source of all diseases" and "all diseases arise from depression" refer to the generality of clinical depression syndrome, which also reveals the generality of psychosomatic causes. Depression syndrome and liver failure usually show the following pathological conditions: Due to certain stimuli (mostly negative frustration, frustration, frustration, willingness failure, sadness, etc.), patients are emotionally depressed, groaning, or sad, or crying, or laughing inconstantly, such as depression, instability; in the body, such as poor appetite, loss of appetite, even anorexia, abdominal distension, nausea and other disorders; and often involuntary. The geographer sighs, sighs a little wide, cold sexual desire, low sexual function; women can still see breast pain, less abdominal pain, is caused by delayed menstruation, not smooth, and so on. Combined with modern clinical practice, when liver fails to govern free flow of qi, it can further lead to cholecystitis, epigastric pain, gastrointestinal dysfunction, arrhythmia, insomnia, headache, elevated blood pressure, etc. Long-term liver failure and drainage may lead to pathological results such as Qi stagnation, phlegm coagulation, blood stasis, and sometimes eventually develop into tumors due to affecting the operation of qi, blood and body fluid.

From the perspective of psychosomatic (physical) medicine or psychiatry, it is not difficult to see that this is actually similar to what is called an atypical, depressive neurosis in modern times. As people live in the real society, emotions or desires often suffer some setbacks, and more importantly, there will be a variety of hidden difficulties, or in times of frustration, failure, and dissatisfaction, which can be interpreted by TCM theory as the "free flow" of the liver is not smooth (the instinctive desire and impulse are repressed). In addition, there are inadequate ability, missed opportunities, and regret, which belong to the liver's inability to free flow; their common result is "the disorder of free flow." This etiology and pathological mechanism prompt a large proportion of people to manifest the above symptoms. Because these conditions are so common that they can occur at any time, or every person may encounter them in his or her life, the clinical symptoms are also very common. The more typical of these diseases can be concluded as "depression syndrome."

In a word, depression has two meanings: one is emotional depression; the other is depression due to loss of qi. All of them are manifested by the internal uncoordinated functions of many viscera, which tend to be weak or disordered. And "depression syndrome" is closely related to liver failure, which is called "universal." Therefore, there are the saying that "depression is the source of all diseases" and "all diseases are born with depression."

In China's unique thinking, as a cause and as a psychopathological mechanism of organic integration. This is a good revelation for such problems that we cannot say clearly today.

2) Social root of multiple depression syndromes

Traditional Chinese medicine has also answered the question of the origin of psychological causes well. We further analyze why "liver governs free flow of qi" was born in the Southern Song Dynasty and was from Zhu Danxi, who switched from Neo-Confucianism to medicine? In this way, we can find the clue. We know that most of the important theories of TCM were established in the period of *The Inner Canon of the Yellow Emperor*, and perhaps only the "liver governs free flow of qi" was formed in the late stage. This is not an accident, but has its own profound social and historical roots.

As we all know, Zhao Xing, Cheng Zhu and other founders founded the Confucian school of idealist philosophy of the Song and Ming dynasties, intended to regulate people's behavior. This action was highly valued by the Song Dynasty and was vigorously implemented. And Neo-Confucianism has a core idea, that is, to "preserve natural principles, destroy human desire." In other words, stemming from the need to maintain feudal rule, these imperial scholars strongly advocated that the various instinctive sexual desires of human beings should be suppressed in order to conform to the supreme "nature." Since then, a whole set of feudal ethics outlines, such as the three outlines and the five constant outlines, have really begun to run wild in China and become the shackles of the behavior of the common people. Neo-Confucianists had also repeatedly advocated that sexual activities such as exquisite appetite and non-reproductive purposes are against the natural principles...

The forcible prohibition of thought and behavior and the excessive repression and repression of instinct soon lead to negative social and health consequences. After entering the Southern Song Dynasty and Yuan and Ming Dynasty, the number of patients with depression syndrome increased dramatically in clinical practice. "Depression" became the precursor of many internal injuries and miscellaneous diseases, so there is the saying that "all diseases arise from depression." It is the fact that physicians in Yuan and Ming Dynasty deeply felt in the clinic that they paid so much attention to the theory of "liver governs free flow of qi," and so focused on the exploration and elaboration of the mechanism of depression syndrome. Relatively speaking, before the Tang Dynasty, the Chinese people's mentality was relatively sound and the living atmosphere was relaxed. So, before Song Dynasty, few physicians discussed such issues as "depression syndrome." It can be seen that social factors thus affect the psychosocial state of social members, thus becoming health or disease problems. The rationality of the "bio-psycho-social medicine" model is also to help people reveal such a profound relationship.

Unfortunately, the negative impact of Neo-Confucianism on the civilian population has remained so far. People often say that Chinese people are implicit, like introspection and self-blame, and stress the word "tolerance" first. This, despite being a behavioral virtue, helps to coordinate human relations, but sometimes also causes people to pay a heavy pathological "cost." That is, they are constantly in a state of depression and discomfort, and liver abnormalities are neglected, which has caused many health and disease pathological problems. It has become a common and important problem that endangers health and Chinese people have to pay enough attention to.

(2) OTHER THEORIES

As for psychopathology, TCM still has many profound insights, such as the theory of seven emotions, personality endowment, which is about the path mechanism of interference with qi, phlegm-generating and blood-stasis, injury to the five viscera, exhaustion of Qi and blood and so on. Since most of them have been well known, textbooks have been introduced in detail, so will not be discussed here.

3.5.7 Prevention of psychological (psychosomatic) diseases

Traditional Chinese medicine is practical. TCM has too much to deal with the theoretical understanding of psychological (psychosomatic) disease prevention. Because the content is too much, here we just enumerate something which people ignore and localization deserves special attention.

(1) PROPOSE MULTIPLE PREVENTIVE RESTRAINT MECHANISMS

Take Zhu Danxi as an example (because the relevant content is too rich, with the characteristics of various schools). In view of the widespread situation of the disorder of free flow of qi, liver depression and qi stagnation caused by the frequent suppression of excessive desire and ministerial fire, Zhu Danxi proposes a set of prevention and restraint mechanisms to control the frequent sprouting (excessive free flow of qi) of desire spirit (ministerial fire), which contains the thought of psychosomatic medicine with Chinese characteristics.

1) "Preserve nature and destroy human desire"
Zhu Danxi learned from Zhu Xi and other Neo-Confucianists in his early years. Zhu Xi put forward such propositions as "human desire," "human mind," "Tao mind" and "nature" in philosophy. The so-called human desire and human mind have similar meanings. The human mind refers to human nature, driven by human desire (desire spirit), often sensed by external things, which is evil and unlimited. "Tao mind" and nature have both relevance and difference: Tao mind refers to the behavioral activities that conform to human ethical principles; nature includes not only social ethical norms such as human ethical principles, but also behaviors that conform to norms, such as feeling hungry and wanting to eat, feeling cold and wanting to get warm, marrying at the marriageable age, which belong to the category of natural principles. So, it can be said that "Tao mind" is subordinate to "nature," which are both kind and limited. But nature and human desire are incompatible as water and fire. "Eat is nature, but demand delicious is human desire." Though both of them are in the act of sustaining the life of the individual and the lineage, one is rational and temperate, the other driven only by the principle of pleasure satisfaction. Therefore, there is no one who mixes nature and human desire together, when the nature survived, the human desire is died, when the human desire is survived, the nature is died. (*Zhu Zi Quotation Part IV*) The purpose of Neo-Confucianism is to "preserve nature and destroy human desires. "Zhu Danxi, who turned from Neo-Confucianism to medicine, naturally inherited the tenet of Neo-Confucianism. He not only fully affirmed the importance of instinctive desire and impulse for life maintenance, but also adhered to the doctrine "preserve nature and destroy human desires," advocated the suppression of non-separable desires such as appetite, sensual pleasures, etc., which are easy to sprout, and in the process of implementing this principle of keeping fit, he carried out his profound elaboration of the relationship between instinct and rationality.

2) "Teach people to bring mind back and nourish their hearts"
Zhu Danxi believed that in order to prevent hyperactivity of ministerial fire and exuberant desire spirit, specific measures to restrain instincts should be "teach people to bring mind back and nourish their hearts." The so-called "bringing mind back" refers to minimizing or avoiding contact with external stimuli such as sound, color, fragrance and so on, "not seeing what you want, keeping your heart free"; that is, reducing the activities of "consciousness." It is best to return to the state of "closing the door" as advocated by *Lao Zi*, so that the mood is quiet, the ministerial fire is not active and the desire spirit is distracted. The so-called "nourishing the heart" has profound meaning. Zhu Danxi yearned for the "saints" living standards described

in *The Inner Canon of the Yellow Emperor* and quoted Zhou Dunyi's saying: "The saints are determined to be just and righteous and claim quiet." That is to say, the Confucian, especially the neo-Confucian (Neo-Confucianism) doctrine is used to edify the "heart" and strengthen its own restraint power, so that it can inherently resist the urge to restrain instinctive desire, that is, self-suppression, weakening the "desire spirit."

3) "The human mind obeys the fate is Tao mind"
On this basis, around the issue of instinct, he further introduced the concepts of "human mind" and "Tao mind" of the Neo-Confucianists, pointing out that "this is ministerial fire. The human mind obeys the life is Tao mind, and it can be quiet primarily. The five fires are all in the middle section. Ministerial fire is only helpful to make up for each other. Zhu Danxi also directly quotes Zhu Xi's saying: "Tao mind must always be the masters of one's body, while human mind obeys their fate." Based on this, he demonstrates his attitude of "adoptive heart" toward instinct (desire spirit). In this way, Zhu Danxi constructed a relatively complete theory system of "instinct."

4) Make good use of bitter cold and know "free flow of ministerial fire"
Perhaps, the imprint of Neo-Confucian is too profound. Zhu believed that many of the above links were still insufficient to control the vigorous and easily delusional instinct ("desire spirit"), so he advocated the use of bitter drugs such as Rhizoma Anemarrhenae and Cortex Phellodendri to "free flow of ministerial fire" and "strengthen kidney." The so-called diarrhea and fire, strengthening the kidney, its meaning lies in the use of biological means to weaken the instinctive desire impulse, reduce kidney refinement and excretion. Both clinical and experimental results show that Cortex Phellodendron can significantly inhibit sexual function, reduce the secretion of related hormones, and affect appetite, which achieves the efficacy of free flow of ministerial fire and suppressing desire spirit (see Figure 3-4).

(2) Cross-cultural comparison between Zhu Danxi and Freud

Perhaps, localization can be more profound through cross-cultural comparison. Therefore, we can use Freund's theory of spiritual structure to analyze the deep meaning of Danxi's theory. Zhu Danxi's "ministerial fire" is similar to the "original self" in Freud's theory, which refers to the motivation of seeking desire satisfaction or "desire spirit," and can also be regarded as the internal drive (vitality) of life; it is mainly related to properties. Zhu's quotation of the "human mind" refers to

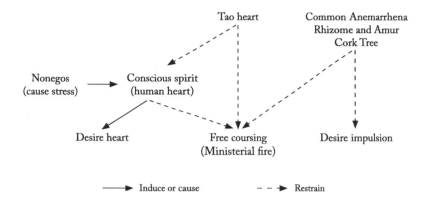

Figure 3-4   Preventive and Restrictive Mechanisms to Control the Frequent Emergence of Desire spirit in Zhu Danxi.

the individual's conscious self-consciousness, and some of the actions resulting therefrom, which are similar to what Freund said of the "self." As for "Tao mind," Zhu Danxi refers to the self-personality and rational force strictly following the social civilization norms recognized by Neo-Confucianist, close to what Freund called "superego." The so-called "human mind obeys the Tao mind" is to make oneself conscious and absolutely obey the set of social ethical norms (natural) advocated by the scientist, so as to achieve the "Tao mind" can dominate all one's own behavior from time to time, including all kinds of instinctive desires and impulses. In addition, the "human mind" can strengthen its own intrinsic inhibitory effect on the Spirit of desire, so as to effectively prevent the danger of the easily sprouting Spirit of desire to the Spirit of origin, including health. It can be seen that Zhu Danxi proposed a three-fold prevention and restraint mechanism to control the frequent sprouting of desire spirits (Ministerial fire): 1) By not seeing what one wants, we can make the mind not disturbed; 2) keeping the mind calm and restraining the ministerial fire; 3) keeping the mind under the control of the Tao, in order to make the Tao mind always the master of the body, that is, strengthening the restraint role of social norms. In addition, the inhibition of drugs constitutes a complete system of understanding, prevention and control of instinct. This system had a great influence at that time. As long as Zhang Jingyue strongly opposed Zhu Danxi's theory of using bitter cold to govern the free flow of ministerial fire more than 200 years later and believed that Zhu's theory had caused the time and disadvantages in the medical field for hundreds of years, and advocated the theory of "true yang," one or two could be seen.

(3) WHY SHOULD WE USE "MINISTERIAL FIRE" LESS IN FUTURE GENERATIONS AND REPLACE IT MORE WITH "FREE FLOW"

After Zhu Shi, physicians in Ming and Qing Dynasty gradually decrease the use of the word "Ministerial fire" to characterize the instinctive desire and impulse, especially after Zhang Jingyue rose his academic and questioned Danxi's "*Theory of Ministerial Fire*," physicians rarely used this word, but gradually borrowed the word "free flow." When we analyze the reasons, there may be two reasons.

(1) The meaning of "free flow" itself includes catharsis, externalization, catharsis, etc. The desire and impulse of human instinct is a kind of vent and expression of potential originating from inside; if it is relaxed, it achieves its purpose, but it does not necessarily have the sign of "fire." Semantically, free flow seems to be more fit than ministerial fire. Free flow also gradually has the same meaning as "desire spirit." Therefore, diet, sexual desire, emotions and so on are all considered to be subject to "free flow." The free flow of "liver" can adjust the Qi movement, thereby regulating emotions, sexual function and diet.

(2) Read the doctrines well, we can see that after the Yuan and Ming dynasties, in many medical books for a time, "ministerial fire" has the naked desire, pornographic characteristics, saying that people "have a strong ministerial fire," undoubtedly emphasizes the strong sexual desire, frequent sexual life. It's too tough. However, physicians who emphasize implicitness and elegance gradually use less such words to refer to more crepe and clever words (free flow), which also seems to be one of the factors behind it.

The localization of clinical psychological application (operation) is more abundant, colorful and practical, which will be described in detail in the future.

Harmonizing the World

Traditional Chinese Medicine and the Thought of "Harmony"
in Chinese Traditional Culture

LECTURER: WANG QINGQI

Introduction to the speaker:

Wang Qingqi, a tenured professor of Shanghai University of Traditional Chinese Medicine and famous traditional Chinese medicine doctor in Shanghai, enjoys the special allowance of the State Council Government. He is a tutor of academic experience inheritance of renowned traditional Chinese medicine doctors in China and also the chief editor of the traditional Chinese medicine subject in *Cihai Dictionary*. He has tutored 40 doctors, post-doctors, and academic inheritors. He has been the editor in chief and deputy editor in chief of more than 50 scholarly works. He has been engaged in clinical medicine (digestive system and psychosomatic diseases) and teaching *The Inner Canon of the Yellow Emperor* for more than 50 years. He has won the first prize in Shanghai Traditional Chinese Medicine's Scientific and Technological Achievements and the second prize of Scientific and Technical Results of the Chinese Academy of Traditional Chinese Medicine. He is also the host of the famous psychological teacher studio of traditional Chinese medicine of Shanghai Education Commission.

4.1 Introduction: Is Traditional Chinese Medicine Scientific?

Difference in profession makes one feel worlds apart. Thus, there may be different views on traditional Chinese medicine in society. Some think it is very mysterious, while some others consider it significant. Furthermore, whether traditional Chinese medicine is scientific or not keeps hitting the headlines and remains to be discussed.

Indeed, traditional Chinese medicine is medicine of Chinese people, a survivor technique for us. Two hundred years before the spread of western medicine to China, Chinese people had to fight against diseases for survival, leading to traditional Chinese medicine. Hu Shi (a thinker known for the New Culture Movement in China) once said, "*What is culture? Culture is a way of survival or a way of life.*" Yu Qiuyu (a Chinese cultural scholar) said, "*Culture is a combination of lifestyle and spiritual value.*" Therefore, Chinese medical culture is our Chinese way of life and survivor technique. Although some people query science of traditional Chinese medicine, I believe the problem does not exist. With a history of thousands of years, the technique is proved useful. There must be scientific elements of valuable things.

Similarly, while Chinese use chopsticks and spoons for meals, westerners use forks and knives. Both serve as survivor techniques for different races and have nothing to do with science. You cannot deem chopsticks unscientific. Otherwise, how can Chinese people survive without this technique? Accordingly, denying traditional Chinese medicine is negating traditional Chinese culture and the way of survival for thousands of years. Traditional Chinese medicine is medicine of Chinese people or our science.

4.2 Philosophy of "Harmony"

Zhang Dainian, one of the most famous modern philosophers and a professor of philosophy at Peking University, said, "*There are two greatest contributions that traditional Chinese culture has made to world civilization. Firstly, the concept of 'heaven-man oneness.' Second, the theory of interpersonal relationships that 'harmony is most precious.'*"

Li Zhonghua, another professor of philosophy at Peking University, said, "*The wisdom of Chinese philosophy is embodied in character 'he' (和, harmony). It is a fundamental spirit and characteristic of Chinese nation and the highest values of Chinese philosophy and culture.*" As the citation from Hu Shi that culture is a way of survival, traditional Chinese culture is Chinese way of survival. "Harmony" is an idea extracted from the direction of survival or culture. In fighting against nature and getting along with each other, our ancestors advocated a culture, that is, "harmony."

For thousands of years, the idea of "harmony" has developed from Confucianism, such as *"to achieve balanced harmony"* and *"to make harmony a top priority in application of rites,"* to today's concept of *"harmonious society."* It has permeated all aspects of Chinese civilization, including philosophy, history, politics, ethics, religion, education, literature, art, etc. Hence the idea has profoundly affected lives of Chinese people. Traditional Chinese medicine is another important field influenced by the idea of "harmony."

4.3   Concepts of "He (和)" in Traditional Chinese Culture

Then let us focus on how the idea of "harmony" is reflected in traditional Chinese medicine. In my research on "harmony," I found two earliest meanings of character "he (和)."

(1) The first meaning of "he (和)" refers to harmony of tunes. The character was originated early from oracle bone inscription "龢 (he)." It is the same as "和 (he)," though most people do not know. The original meaning of "龢 (he)" is tuning, that is, to produce beautiful music through blending various rhymes in a moderate range. As is mentioned in *Yue Ji*, *"When appreciating music, gentlemen enjoy sonority and grasp the idea of harmony (合, he)."* That is to say, when we listen to music by a gentleman – an ideally right person in ancient times, as opposed to base persons – we should admire both sonorous sounds and harmonious blend. Character "合 (he)" is true "和 (he)." The more harmonious notes are, the more pleasant music may be. This is the primary meaning of "he (和)."

(2) The second meaning of "he (和)" refers to harmony of wines. Wine was invented early since the origin of Chinese culture. The traditional Chinese form of character "医 (yi, medicine)" is 醫 (yi), with a "酉 (you)" at the bottom, meaning wine. Then how did traditional Chinese medicine begin? For one thing, it is a summary of Chinese experience in fighting against diseases. The earliest therapy is to soak medicinal herbs in wine and make it a medicated wine, which is the first Chinese medicinal preparation. For another, traditional Chinese medicine is a harmonious combination of various medicinal flavors according to specific rules, to exert its therapeutic effect. The decoction we drink was invented by Yi Yin, a chef who needs seasoning. The seasoning is nothing more than oil, salt, sauce, and vinegar, but a high-level chef can bring out delicious dishes. Similarly, several dozen medicines in a formula need to be combined according to different flavors and efficacy for better effect.

Later, the meaning of "he (和)" was extended to a reasonable yardstick of behavior and unified coordination of multiple elements. For instance, we have heart, liver, spleen, lungs, and kidneys in our body. "he (和)" coordinates various viscera. "He (和)" means healthy and normal, while not "he (和)" means abnormal. Another example is that we have 56 ethnic groups in China. Most ethnic groups have their lifestyle, culture, customs, and writing. If all ethnic groups want to live together in harmony, it implies unified coordination of multiple elements. Therefore, the meaning of "he (和)" has been extended from tuning and seasoning.

4.4 Development of "Harmony" in Literature before The Inner Canon of the Yellow Emperor

Book of Rites says, "*Music of a peaceful society is pleasant, indicating stable politics; music of a chaotic society is resenting, indicating turbulent politics; music of a conquered nation is sorrowful, indicating suffering of its people.*" Music is used to describe whether society is harmonious or not. Peaceful music is beautiful. "Stable politics" suggests that decrees can be carried out smoothly in a harmonious society. On the contrary, "turbulent politics" indicates that the community is inharmonious because of fighting and confusion, not a sight of prosperous state and peaceful people.

Book of History is the earliest compilation of political documents in our country, known as central literature. It records a few situations of political life in the Western Zhou Dynasty. Focusing on "harmonizing the world," the book established a system of norms on "harmony." Specific instructions include: "Harmony" is a requirement and principle of governance; "harmony" is a method and standard for management; "harmony" is a demand for bureaucratic relations, family relationships, and brotherhood.

Book of Changes is the first Chinese philosophical work. It was finished in the Spring and Autumn Period, with Confucius allegedly participating in writing. The yin-yang theory and five-phase theory in traditional Chinese medicine originated from *The Book of Changes*. There are many records of hexagrams in the book. Each hexagram contains three parts: "proper position," "corresponding position," and "median position." Hexagrams are used to foretell the future according to these three parts, reflecting a pursuit of "balanced harmony." Therefore, some scholars believe that *Book of Changes* adhered to "advocating balanced harmony" from cover to cover.

Discourses on Governance of the States was written in the later Spring and Autumn Period and the Warring States Period. It puts forward several ideas, including "differentiation between harmony and uniformity," "seeking harmony in differences," and "harmony begets new things, while uniformity does not lead to continuation." As is mentioned, "harmony" is unity of various things. "Uniformity" is accumulation of the same elements. Therefore, "harmony" is different from "uniformity." "Harmony" means coexistence, reflecting relationships among two or more objects. "Uniformity" only means accumulation of one single purpose. "Harmony begets new things" indicates that only when multiple diverse things coexist in harmony can new ideas be produced. For example, a man belongs to yang, and a woman belongs to yin. "*Harmony of yin and yang contributes to birth of children.*" A man and a woman can harmoniously combine for reproduction.

Similarly, things of yang can organically combine with things of yin to produce new things. For example, heaven belongs to yang, and earth belongs to yin. When heaven qi rises, and earth qi falls, yin and yang intersect, resulting in evolution of wind, rain, thunder, and lightning. "Dog days" means precisely the season when earth qi rises and heaven qi falls. Hence, intersection of yin and yang leads to particularly hot weather in summer and many unpredictable natural phenomena. "*Uniformity does not lead to continuation*" means addition of the same things only contributes to an increase in quantity but has no effect on creating new things. Thus, combination of things with the same properties cannot beget anything new. The simplest example is that two men cannot procreate. The opinion that there is no philosophy in China is wrong because we can see from old sayings that traditional Chinese culture is full of philosophy. "*Harmony begets new things*" reflects the importance of "harmony." Only "harmony" can continuously produce and evolve new things. If relationships between colleagues in a company are in discord, work efficiency may be low, hindering tasks' smooth progress. If people with different knowledge structures are grouped to form a unit, the unit will become a joint force to promote development, which well interprets "harmony begets new things." Similar phenomena abound in the colorful world. "Uniformity does not lead to continuation" only results in decay and extinction.

Tao Te Ching, a classic by Lao Tzu, was also finished in the Spring and Autumn Period. It says, "*Everything bears yin and embraces yang. Harmony derives from intersection of yin qi and yang qi.*" It means things in the boundless universe can be divided into yin and yang, which can be integrated harmoniously. "Intersection of yin qi and yang qi" shows heaven qi interacts with earth qi. "Harmony" is a natural state of all things in the world. All things inherently contain factors of yin and yang. Yin qi and yang qi from internal and external sides depend on and originate from each other and oppose each other. Thus, all things maintain a state of "convergence." The ancients also used the yin-yang theory to explain earthquakes. They believed underground energy would burst out when it accumulated to a certain extent. Then interaction between yin and yang in the process could produce an earthquake. The theory can also be applied to weather. Yin qi interacts with yang qi to produce wind, rain, thunder, and lightning. Too much interaction results in natural disasters, while harmony means a regular weather pattern. The ancients used the theory to interpret both natural and social phenomena. Lao Tzu also said, "*To soften the light and accept the dust.*" Light represents heaven, and dust represents earth. Humans should live with heaven and earth (Nature), emphasizing the idea of "harmony."

Analects of Confucius is work during the Spring and Autumn Period and the Warring States Period. It is said that Confucius had visited Lao Tzu, who was a few years older than Confucius. When Confucius was in his twenties, Lao Tzu was already in his forties. It says in the book, "*Make harmony a top priority in application of rites. This is a key feature that characterizes governance by sovereign rulers in the ancient past. Always act upon rules of harmony, no matter whether the issue is minor or major.*" It means that the crux of rites is to handle minor and major things to a right point.

Rites are used to regulate people's behavior. Rules of rituals in ancient times are the same as rules of law today. Therefore, Confucius proposed restoring control of rites in the Zhou Dynasty governed by Duke of Zhou. He believed country and society would be in a muddle without it. Then how to regulate people's behavior? We should make harmony a top priority. Law should be combined with a spirit of "harmony" to deal with different matters. The book also puts forward a gentleman spirit of "*being harmonious yet different.*" In chapter *Zi Lu*, it writes, "*Gentlemen are in harmony with each other despite differences between them, whereas base persons are in disharmony with each other despite uniformity among them.*" Base persons are not villains. In the realm of ideology, a gentleman is an ideal talent, whereas base persons have narrower horizons. Thus, perfect gentlemen should follow the concept of "being harmonious yet different." In a company, workers should get along in harmony despite differences. Business will flourish if everyone not only shows his strengths but also cooperates to make joint efforts. However, base persons are harmonious on the surface but intrigue against each other behind the backs. Thus, the idea of "being harmonious yet different" has become a spiritual beacon that guides Chinese "literati" class to think independently and behave with integrity for thousands of years.

Doctrine of the Mean writes, "*What heaven has bestowed upon people is called human nature. Acting following this moral nature is called Tao (the way).*" "*Balance is a foundation under heaven, while harmony is a universal rule under heaven.*" That is, the way under heaven is to achieve harmony. Balance means impartiality. Only with justice can there be harmony. Thus, in words "to achieve balanced harmony," "balanced" and "harmony" are inseparable. Also, the book also writes, "*Both heaven and earth will be in their proper places, and all things will prosper and thrive.*" "Both heaven and earth will be in their proper places" mean if "balanced harmony" is achieved, "*everything will have its position and grow well.*" If everyone in a company sticks to his post, business will flourish. And it is the same in Nature. In Shanghai, there is a high school called "Wei Yu." "Wei" means "place" and "Yu," says "thrive." The name originated from the sentence above, aiming to cultivate students who can do their jobs well and thus help society produce high energy.

Mo Tzu was finished a little later. It advocates "exalting the worthy," that is, to respect, promote, and employ worthy and able men in governance regardless of origin and intimacy. Mo Tzu had great insights into governance, which is worth emulation. Moreover, he also put forward the concept of "conforming upwardly (unity)." He thought the cause of chaos in the state and disharmony among father, son, and brothers was disunity of "righteousness." Therefore, "conforming upwardly" is not a dictatorship, but so-called "harmony." For instance, instead of making a final decision on his own, the emperor should solicit opinions widely. The concept of "conforming upwardly" emphasizes that only a harmonious country and society can develop well.

Mencius and *Xunzi* can be classified into Confucianism. The two books put forward opposite opinions as to human nature. *Mencius* writes, "*Man on earth, good at birth.*" Experiences will encroach innate kindness in society, so receiving an education is necessary. On the contrary, *Xunzi* says human nature is evil and selfish. People should receive training from family, society, and school to improve their quality and become talents. Despite some different views, both books belong to Confucianism, which takes a fundamental stand that "harmony of people" contributes to making a great country. Mencius believed that governors should value "harmony of people," which can "achieve popular support all under heaven" and thus build "a secure country and a powerful army." In *Mencius, Gong Sun Chou II*, it says, "*Favorable weather conditions are not as valuable as favorable geographic conditions, and favorable geographic conditions are not as valuable as harmony of people.*" In brief, "harmony of people" is far more critical than "harmony" of time or space.

Xunzi considered "harmony of people" as an important condition for "a prosperous country" and "a powerful ruler." In governance, there are benevolence and hegemony. Benevolence means democracy, that is, to win over people by ideological work. Hegemony means rules of law, that is, to regulate people's behavior with laws. The idea of benevolence and hegemony is also reflected in combination and formulas of traditional Chinese medicine. That is because principles of governance, human relationship, and health preservation were consistent in ancient China.

In *Xunzi, Wang Ba*, it says, "*If favorable weather conditions, geographic advantages, and people's harmony are all obtained, Everything will be in progress. Policies will be smoothly carried out, and customs will be pleasantly observed. Under such circumstances, guard can be strengthened, and enemies can be defeated. People can earn a good reputation inside and achieve merits outside.*" It means favorable time, space, and people's harmony can help implement various policies effectively throughout the country, contributing to a prosperous state with peaceful people.

Master Lü's Spring and Autumn Annals, edited by Lü Buwei, is another representative work of Confucianism. Classified as syncretism, the book is so inclusive that it collects Confucianism, Taoism, Legalism, Mohism, Logicianism, philosophy of School of Military, and yin-yang theory, etc. Lü thinks that "Tai Yi (oneness)" is the origin of all things. "*Tai Yi produces Liang Yi (duality), and Liang Yi produces yin and yang. With yang moves upward and yin downward, they integrate and produce Everything.*" More specifically, "*In the beginning, heaven was formed by rising, slight substances, and earth was composed of falling heavy matters. Integration of heaven and earth is the source of Everything.*" To put it bluntly, "Tai Yi" is universe, and "Liang Yi" is heaven and earth. Heaven belongs to yang, and earth belongs to yin. When yin and yang integrate, all things exist. This is both a philosophical idea and an outlook that explains how the world is formed, how Everything is produced, and how life is created. Although "Tai Yi" is the origin of all things, its function of generating ideas is performed by interaction and integration of yin (earth) and yang (heaven). After creation, Everything must depend on the nourishing of yin qi, yang qi, rain, and dew to grow. This is the interpretation of "Tai yin produces Liang Yi," which emphasizes that "harmony is the way of heaven, with which everything can exist and thrive."

To summarize, "harmony" is an outlook and methodology of Confucianism. It regards impartiality and balance as the highest moral standard and fundamental principle of handling things. "Harmony" has two meanings. One refers to "harmony begets new things." As *Xunzi* writes, "*Everything obtains its harmony to grow and nourishment to mature.*" The other refers to "being harmonious yet different." It means unity of diversity can enrich, develop, create new things, and form a colorful world. "Being harmonious yet different" reflects great wisdom of human ideals. Our worlds should be the same global village under the same universe, so we should advocate the idea.

4.5   The Thought of "Harmony" in Inner Canon of the Yellow Emperor

Traditional Chinese medicine and Chinese traditional culture are derived from the same origin. Chinese medicine is an integral part of China's traditional culture. Chairman Xi Jinping said: "Chinese medicine is the key to open the treasure house of Chinese civilization." Some people say that there is no philosophy in China. We all learn from a different philosophy, which is wrong, so we should start the revitalization of Chinese from the revival of Chinese culture. Although you don't study traditional Chinese medicine, you can understand it. I'm here to promote it. Traditional Chinese medicine and traditional culture are derived from the same origin. If we deny traditional Chinese medicine, we will reject the whole traditional culture.

The word "Harmony" appeared 159 times in *The Inner Canon of the Yellow Emperor*, and "Harmony" is a critical core concept, or core values, in the theoretical construction of traditional Chinese medicine. The original meaning of "Harmony" is to maintain and restore body's self-regulation mechanism. There are all kinds of substances in human body, which can coordinate the functions of yin and yang, nutrient-defense, Qi and blood, body fluids, zang-fu organs, and other systems to maintain normal physiological activities. They are not assembled like machines but are combined harmoniously. A watch is assembled with small parts. It has no life, but human beings have. Only when all kinds of substances are combined harmoniously can vitality of experience be produced. This is "Harmony."

By learning the thought of "Harmony" in traditional Chinese medicine, we can not only fully learn from ancients' wisdom to resolve those crisis between man and nature, man and society, man and himself brought by the thought of "binary opposition" in the development of modern society, but also deeply understand the thinking mode of traditional Chinese medicine. If you want to follow traditional Chinese medicine, first of all, you need to understand the culture of traditional Chinese medicine, further understand how traditional Chinese medicine doctor treats illness, how to appreciate nature, human body physiology, and pathology. To say, to understand the thinking mode of traditional Chinese medicine, which originates from traditional culture. Therefore, we need to grasp the essence of traditional Chinese medicine and improve the practical level of traditional Chinese medicine, to provide useful help to solve the problems of prevention and treatment of chronic non-infectious diseases and new infectious diseases faced in modern medicine, to correct the disadvantages of confrontation treatment and overtreatment, to correct the wrong understanding of doctor-patient relationship, and to ease the contradictions between doctors and patients. We can use the idea of "harmony" to interpret those problems when correcting the current gap between Chinese and Western medicine and the contradictions between doctors and patients.

Western medicine published the definition of health in 1945, which considered three standards of health, including that body doesn't get ill, mind is healthy, and can adapt to society well. This definition is universally accepted. What does *The Inner Canon of the Yellow Emperor* say about health? *Miraculous Pivot · Ben Zang* said: "Therefore, Harmony of blood and Qi will make the meridians unobstructed. To spread nutrition throughout the whole body, make muscles and bones strong, and to male joints smooth." Blood is an essential component of human body. Seven-tenths of human body is liquid, and a large part of the liquid is blood. Blood continually flows in human body, "blood harmony" means that blood usually flows, and body is good. Traditional Chinese medicine is about Qi and blood. Qi is an invisible and primary material to maintain human life. How? Qi also continually flows into human body. "Qi harmony" means the smooth movement of Qi. "Harmony of defense Qi will make the muscles stretch, and smooth, the skin soft and harmonious in color, the striae and interstice is close together." The striae and interstice mean the sweat hole, which is like a door with the opening and closing function. When it is hot, it will open and sweat. When it is cold, it will close. Who is in charge of this gate? It's the defense Qi. "Harmony of will and ideation will make the essence-spirit concentrate, and straight, ethereal soul and human soul will not disperse. The resentment and anger will not attack, so the five viscera will not be disturbed by external evil. Harmony of clod and warm will make the six bowels digest the grain normally so that moving impediment will not occur, the meridians will be unblocked, and the movement of limbs and joints will be safe and normal. These are the normal physiological states of human body." This means that people, as long as they have these conditions, are healthy.

To sum up, the essence of health is harmony. What are the aspects of harmony? Harmony between coldness and warmness, qi and blood, and between the will and ambition.

"Harmony of coldness and warmness" is Harmony of man and nature. "Harmony of will and ideation" is Harmony of mind and body, physiology, and psychology; "Harmony of qi and blood" is Harmony of human body's internal environment. Mr. Ji Xianlin once appointed the meaning of "harmony," has three aspects. The first point is Harmony between man and nature, the second point is Harmony between man and man, and the third point is Harmony between the heart and body. Mr. Ji Xianlin's view is the same as that of our traditional Chinese medicine. In a word, health is a harmonious state between human and nature, physiology and psychology, qi, and blood. "Healthy" is a state, which continually changes. It exists in the process from birth to death. Human body state continually changes. It may change from a healthy state to a sub-healthy state, then to an unhealthy state, more to a disease state, and finally to death. There have been changes in human and nature, physiology and psychology, qi and blood, these three aspects in this process.

So, what is a disease? Human body is a large system; each system has its own unique function. There should be numerous contradictory and unified contradictions in human body, such as Yin and Yang, Qi and blood, viscera and bowels, exterior and interior, water and fire, ascending and descending, dynamic and static, exhalation and inhalation, generation and restriction, the element is restricted and unrestricted, etc. The simplest example is exhaling and inhaling. People inhale oxygen and emit carbon dioxide, which is a pair of contradictions. To handle this, human body has its self-regulation system, which is called "harmful hyperactivity and responding inhibition" in *The Inner Canon of the Yellow Emperor*. This is a kind of regulatory capacity. If you sneeze repeatedly, it's a sign that you're cold and sick. But when you get sick, you don't have to go to the hospital, because body can self-regulate. You can drink some boiled water and sleep the next day. However, people with weak resistance still need to see a doctor because of their poor self-regulation ability.

Western medicine believes that disease is human body's response to environmental stimuli, which is the sum of organisms' abnormal responses to abnormal stimuli. Bacteria, viruses, physical factors, chemical factors, and all kinds of dust are pathogenic factors. After being stimulated, human body will make an abnormal reaction, and this is disease. If you have excellent resistance, you will be able to "bear the burden of excessive harm" and be able to self-control; but some people can't, and they have to see a doctor for emergency treatment. Therefore, disease is an unhealthy state of human body. It is a state of disharmony between man and nature, the discord of mind and body, and the disharmony of qi and blood. *The Inner Canon of the Yellow Emperor* said: "Blood and Qi disharmony, all diseases are caused by changes." This is a classic generalization.

The Inner Canon of the Yellow Emperor said: "Qi harmonizes with each other to get healthy. If Qi is not harmonious with each other, one will get sick." Traditional Chinese medicine believes that Qi in body is constantly running, and the regular operation is healthy while the abnormal operation will get sick. Mr. Feng Youlan is a philosopher at Peking University. In his new edition of *The History of Chinese Philosophy*, he interprets *The Inner Canon of the Yellow Emperor* as a philosophical work because many of its explanations are philosophical.

Qi harmonizes with each other to get healthy. If qi is not harmonious with each other, there are many TCM treatment methods, among which the most classic and the most principled way is "harmonize the disharmony." Disease is the disharmony between heaven and man, heart and body, qi and blood, showing symptoms and reactions, so treatment should be aimed at all kinds of discord. Zhang Jingyue, a medical expert in Ming Dynasty, said: "The medicine for harmonizing prescriptions is also for those who are not in harmony with them. For those who have both deficiency and disease, they should be treated with tonifying and harmonizing them." Harmony is a broad sense, and it is also like soil and four qi. It can be used in reinforcing, reducing, warming and cooling. It is essential to keep a balance of vitality. "Zhang Jingyue also said: "The so-called regulation means to regulate those unregulated." "Where there is no positive Qi" – not correct is called evil, TCM called evil, "We all rely on harmony, such as evil Qi on surface. Expelling is also regulation." Cold, sneezing, coughing, sore throat, this is the reaction of evil Qi on surface, drinking some ginger soup or taking some sweating medicine can expelling evil qi, called "Expelling is also regulation." "If evil qi is inside body, it is necessary to adjust it." If evil qi is inside, oily food should be poured out. "Stagnation of excess and evil, diarrhea is regulation." Yesterday, too much meat and fishy food were eaten, and the stomach was bloated. This morning, my stomach was not hungry. At this time, "diarrhea means regulating," so the stomach's indigestible food was quickly solved. "When you are tired, tonifying means regulating." A person is extremely weak and has no strength at all. He is exhausted and has a deficiency of both qi and Yin. "Tonifying is regulating." Take some medicine for tonifying qi and nourishing yin.

Cheng Zhongling defined "harmony" as one of "eight methods of medicine" in *The Experience of Medicine*. He summarized the treatment principles as follows: "To harmonize, we can clear it, warm it, dissipate it, complement it, dry it, moist it, make people sweat, or even attack it to achieve the goal. The meaning of harmony is one, and the methods of harmony is endless." There are a variety of treatment methods, can be summed up in one word, that is, "to harmonize."

4.6   "Harmony" Thought in Health Preservation

In fact, the principle of "harmony" is also stressed in the aspect of health preservation. There are three health standards: harmony between man and nature, Harmony of mind and body, and harmony of qi and blood. Health maintenance is Harmony of these three aspects. The narrow sense of health preservation, I understand it refers to the maintenance and care of life when there is no disease. Through this maintenance and care, we can achieve the purpose of health and longevity. In a broad sense, health preservation includes the treatment of diseases when they are ill.

I have five views on health preservation.

(1) In fact, health preservation is a kind of mentality that determines health, which is very important. Health preservation aims to prevent and control the occurrence of diseases, which reflects a sense of anxiety.

(2) Health care embodies the love of life.

(3) The principle of health preservation is to maintain Harmony between heaven and man, heart and body, qi, and blood.

(4) The essence of health preservation is to develop healthy and scientific living habits. Health preservation is to develop a good practice, which is conducive to harmony between heaven and man, mind and body, and Qi and blood.

(5) The highest state of health preservation is to forget both the surroundings and even ourselves, following nature, being at ease in mind and body, and being healthy in form and spirit.

4.7   The Cultural Value and Practical Significance of "Harmony"

Chinese philosophical wisdom concentrates on the word "harmony." It is the basic spirit and characteristics of Chinese nation and the highest value standard of Chinese philosophy and Chinese culture. "Harmony" is a kind of value. Ancient books say: "The beauty of heaven and earth lies in harmony," and "harmony" is the most beautiful. *Tao Te Ching* says: "The way of saints is not to fight for," "the way of heaven is to win without fighting," "The only way for a man is not to fight, so the world can not compete with it," which embodies the idea of "harmony." According to the understanding of Chinese philosophy, "struggle" is only surface truth of contradiction, "harmony" is the deep essence of disagreement. The wisdom and outlet of human beings lie in finding the road and understanding how to reconcile contradictions. The practical significance of the concept of "harmony" of Chinese nation or the philosophy of harmony lies in its ability to resolve and rectify various crises caused by the fundamental contradiction of human existence and development, to make it move forward along the road of rational wisdom embodying "harmony but different."

Russell, a Western philosopher, said: "Some of China's supreme ethical qualities are extremely needed in the modern world. Of these qualities, I think amity comes first. "If the world can adopt it, there will certainly be more joy and peace on earth than it is now."

The social value of "harmony" can be summarized as follows.

(1) The thought of "harmony" can promote harmony between man and nature.

(2) The thought of "harmony" can promote Harmony of the individual body and mind.

(3) The thought of "harmony" can improve Harmony between people and society.

(4) The thought of "harmony" can promote world peace.

LECTURE 5

Benefit by Associating Together

Physique and Temperament

LECTURER: WANG QINGQI

Introduction to the speaker:

Wang Qingqi, a tenured professor of Shanghai University of Traditional Chinese Medicine and famous traditional Chinese medicine doctor in Shanghai, enjoys the special allowance of the State Council Government. He is a tutor of academic experience inheritance of renowned traditional Chinese medicine doctors in China and also the chief editor of the traditional Chinese medicine subject in *Cihai Dictionary*. He has tutored 40 doctors, post-doctors, and academic inheritors. He has been the editor in chief and deputy editor in chief of more than 50 scholarly works. He has been engaged in clinical medicine (digestive system and psychosomatic diseases) and teaching *The Inner Canon of the Yellow Emperor* for more than 50 years. He has won the first prize in Shanghai Traditional Chinese Medicine's Scientific and Technological Achievements and the second prize of Scientific and Technical Results of the Chinese Academy of Traditional Chinese Medicine. He is also the host of the famous psychological teacher studio of traditional Chinese medicine of Shanghai Education Commission.

5.1 Reasons for Choosing "Constitution and Temperament" as the Theme of Speech

In daily life or clinic, it is often found that if a person suffers from cold, some people will get sick while others will not. The reason for this may be that people who do not get sick are not easy to get sick because of their good constitution and strong resistance. This is a very simple answer, which shows that people's constitution has a great relationship with the onset of disease or not.

As medical staffs, we also found another phenomenon, for example, when doing a physical examination, some people take a chest X-ray and find there is a calcification. The doctor said that you had tuberculosis, but the patient said that I never had tuberculosis. In fact, this person did get tuberculosis, which healed already, calcification is just the traces after tuberculosis healed. Others may develop symptoms of low fever and bloody coughing after having tuberculosis. Before the introduction of streptomycin, rifampicin, isoniazid and other anti-tuberculosis drugs into China, few people could be cured of tuberculosis.

Both have tuberculosis. Some people heal themselves after they get sick, but others' disease may develop to pulmonary cavities and even endanger their lives. What does this mean? The essence behind these phenomena is the problem of constitution. Constitution determines the tendency and type of the disease. The tendency of disease is like the example of cold mentioned above. Some people get sick while some people do not. The type of diseases varies, as the second example of tuberculosis shows that some people have a very mild onset and heal without feeling anything; others are more typical and develop into refractory diseases later. For example, Among patients infected with SARS, some people feel like catch a cold, heal after taking a little traditional Chinese medicine for two or three days, while others' situation are so severe that they suffer from respiratory failure that they need a lot of hormones, organ cannulation, but maybe still die at last.

We will inevitably encounter unsatisfactory things in our life, or natural and man-made disasters, such as earthquakes. Some people are very unlucky. Their family members died in the earthquake, but they didn't die. As a result, they are worried about the death of their family members and suffer from depression over time. Others, although their family members also die, feeling sad as well, but one or two years later, with the help of the government or the care of relatives and friends, they have recovered well, rebuilt their homes and started a new life, without too much depression. Both suffered natural and man-made disasters, why did one get depression while the other recovered? This is the difference of psychological temperament. People with different psychological temperament have different bearing capacity for natural disasters and man-made disasters and response to various events in daily life.

All the above phenomena show that whether it is the tendency or the type of the disease, it is the constitution that plays a role behind it. Today we are going to discuss the issue of constitution.

5.2   Definition of constitution and temperament

(1) CONSTITUTION

What is constitution? I'm afraid few people can answer. In medical practice and life practice, I found that constitution and temperament play an important role in our mental and physical health.

In ancient Chinese medical literature, there are some records that call it "natural-ability," "natural-ity" and "natural-disposition." It was not until the Qing Dynasty that the word "constitution" really appeared. Therefore, the ancient literature had not seriously explained what is constitution and temperament. Now I will interpret the concept of constitution in English.

The concept of constitution has different interpretations in different disciplines. Modern western medicine defines constitution as follows: constitution is a special state formed gradually in the process of growth and development on the basis of heredity, with relatively stable morphological structure and metabolic function. This is what Professor Kuang Tiaoyuan, an expert in Constitution Research in our university, explained about the concept. This explanation answers two questions:

1)   How is constitution formed? In the first half of the sentence, "constitution is based on heredity," which is the first reason of constitution formation – "heredity"; the second reason is "gradually formed in the process of growth and development." Therefore, the formation of constitution can be summed up in two words, namely "congenital" and "acquired."

2)   What does constitution contain? Constitution includes two aspects of "morpho-logical structure and metabolic function." That is to say, constitution is a state. The state of the body is manifested in two aspects: one is morphological struc-ture. For example, some people are more than 2 meters tall and some are short. This is called constitution, which also belongs to constitution. Foreign countries call constitution. Constitution is also a part of constitution. Generally, people look similar, but they are different.

Physical experts say that just like no two leaves in the world are exactly the same, everyone in the world has different physical fitness. Even identical twins have different physical fitness. Maybe some people think every leaf is the same, but it's not the same. I have consulted experts in plant physiology. I asked him if the plants have physical fitness. He said that different plants have different physical fitness. I thought later that he was right. For example, our traditional Chinese medicine is also a plant. Sichuan's safflower is called Sichuan safflower, and Tibet's safflower is called safflower. All of them are safflower, but one grows in Sichuan and the other grows in Tibet. The price of Tibet is high, and the price of Sichuan is low. Why are the prices different? Because the quality is different, the efficacy is different. It can be seen that all living things, whether plants or animals, have physical problems. Not only human beings have physical problems, but also non-human animals have physical problems. Everyone's physical fitness is different.

"The characteristics of the fertilized egg determine all the properties and functions of the individual," but "it is closely related to the acquired factors, and the constitution is the alloy of the genetic and acquired characteristics of the body." Heredity is inborn, acquisitiveness is acquired. The combination of inborn and acquired forms constitution. When a person is born, he first gets his parents' inborn genes, information and codes; after he is born, he is influenced by the living environment, climate, economic conditions, education, what disease he has suffered in the process of growing up and other factors, forming a different constitution. Therefore, physical fitness is not only related to the genetic code information of parents, but also related to the process of postnatal growth and development.

(2) TEMPERAMENT

Most people don't know what temperament is, so what is temperament? According to modern psychology, temperament is mainly manifested in the intensity, speed and flexibility of psychological activities. It is a relatively stable psychological characteristic of personality. It is related to heredity. It is formed on the basis of people's physiological quality, through life practice and the influence of the day after tomorrow. Therefore, just like constitution, temperament is formed gradually in the acquired living environment on the basis of congenital inheritance. However, temperament is shown as the psychological characteristics of relatively stable individuals such as manner, consciousness, words and deeds, demeanor, which can also be called traits or characteristics. That is, temperament is a state, but also a trait. From the point of view of molecular genetics, temperament is the manifestation of high-level neural activity type in human behavior, and the type of high-level neural activity is the physiological basis of human temperament, which is what Pavlov's advanced neural activity theory tells us. In other words, temperament is not an abstract concept, but has its material basis, which is the type of advanced neural activity. Temperament is the phenomenon of high-level neural activity type in psychological characteristics.

TCM literature records Bing Qi, Bing property and so on. In fact, it refers to temperament, because there were no "constitution" and "temperament" in ancient times.

(3) SIMILARITIES AND DIFFERENCES BETWEEN CONSTITUTION AND TEMPERAMENT

What are the similarities and differences between constitution and temperament? Their similarities are the result of congenital and acquired joint action; the difference is that constitution focuses on physiological function, because body structure and physiological function emphasize physiological function, while temperament focuses on psychological function. Temperament in the formation process, is also affected by congenital genetic factors and acquired environmental factors, but different from physical fitness, acquired factors are more important to the formation of temperament, so temperament plasticity is greater. The formation of constitution is mainly determined by the congenital factors, and related to the acquired factors, but it is inferior to the congenital. Temperament is more dependent on the acquired education, growth environment, contact with the crowd, family environment and so on.

5.3 Characteristics of constitution theory in traditional Chinese Medicine

The records of constitution and temperament in traditional Chinese medicine began from *The Inner Canon of the Yellow Emperor*. The problems of constitution and temperament were discussed in several articles, such as *Divine Pivot · Yinyang 25 people* and *Divine Pivot · Tongtian*, although the words "constitution" and "temperament" did not appear. *The Inner Canon of the Yellow Emperor* contains the concept of "harmony of body and spirit," which is influenced by traditional culture. "Body" is the material basis of "spirit," and "spirit" is the external manifestation of the function of "form." Therefore, traditional Chinese medicine emphasizes the unity of body and spirit, while western medicine advocated separation of body and spirit in the past. This is the difference between traditional Chinese medicine and Western medicine. When it comes to constitution and temperament in *The Inner Canon of the Yellow Emperor*, there are both physical and temperament problems in the behaviors described, which are mixed together. This is not because the ancients were stupid, but influenced by the thought of "unity of body and spirit."

According to this principle, *The Concept of Constitution of Traditional Chinese Medicine* was defined by Professor Wang Qi and I. The concept of constitution in traditional Chinese medicine is described as follows: Constitution refers to a relatively stable special state in terms of morphological structure, physiological function and psychological state formed on the basis of congenital endowment and acquired.

According to the concept of constitution in traditional Chinese medicine, where is the manifestation of constitution? The specific manifestations of constitution are:

a) The morphological characteristics are different. Morphological characteristics are not only manifested in appearance, such as height, but also in the structure of internal organs. Everyone's heart, liver, spleen, lung and kidney may look the same, but in fact they are different, because their physiological functions are different.

b) Physiological and psychological characteristics and reactivity are not the same. For example, there are two brothers. One of them has a good appetite and is very fat and strong; the other has a bad appetite since childhood. They are all born to the same parent, which is the difference in physiological function. One has a very good quality of sleep every day, the other is always unable to sleep, love to ponder, always feels worried. This is the psychological characteristics are not the same. Reactivity refers to the response to external stimuli. For example, when the weather is cold, one is in good health and never gets sick. The other one sneezes, coughs, or has allergies, colds, pneumonia and asthma, and has different responses to external stimuli.

c) The ability to adapt to the environment is different. The environment includes the natural environment and social environment. For example, when foreigners come to Shanghai to study, the natural environment has changed, so has the social environment. Shanghai has its unique natural climate characteristics and human and social environment. Those who live and grow up in the north will feel cold in winter and hot in summer when they arrive in Shanghai. Some people can adapt to these changes, while others can't. People who can adapt to the natural environment have good adaptability; those who can't adapt to the natural environment have poor adaptability, which is the incompatibility between man and nature. The discordance of social environment is reflected in the disharmony of human relations. Outsiders may feel that people in Shanghai are difficult to get along with and can not adapt to the social environment of Shanghai, which is a manifestation of psychological temperament. After living in Shanghai for five years or ten years, they may have adapted to the climatic characteristics of Shanghai and become accustomed to the sweet food in Shanghai. They can also be integrated into the culture of Shanghai people, the actions of Shanghai people and the social environment of Shanghai people. This shows that their constitution and temperament have changed with the change of environment.

d) Resistance to disease is different. For example, epidemics, cold waves, SARS and bird flu are coming. People with strong constitution are not easy to get sick, so they can add a piece of clothes; while weak people will have fever and sneezing, some will become pneumonia, some will have to be hospitalized, and some will even be life-threatening. It's a physical difference.

The above four aspects are the specific manifestation of constitution, specifically, can be summarized as follows.

(1) Susceptibility to some pathogenic factors. In our daily life, we often hear that some people say it's OK to be hot in summer, but we can't stand it in winter, such as asthma and cold. Some people say that it's too hot in summer, and it's quite suitable in winter. Heat and cold, in the view of traditional Chinese medicine, are pathogenic factors, and their susceptibility to each person is different. From the perspective of Western medicine, viruses are pathogenic factors, such as SARS, avian influenza, Zika and other viral microorganisms. Some people infected with the virus is OK, even with the patient contact also does not matter; some people can not, this is caused by different susceptibility to pathogenic factors.

(2) The pathological tendency was different. For example, in the case of Mycobacterium tuberculosis that I mentioned earlier, some people get tuberculosis, but they don't feel it, they don't have any symptoms, they don't need any treatment. After five years and ten years, they have become calcified foci. Some people get tuberculosis, can cough, get low fever, hematemesis, and even appear pulmonary cavity, this is the manifestation of the disease. One does not need to treat themselves, while the other will die without treatment. This indicates that the same disease has different pathological tendency for different people.

(3) The process and prognosis of the disease are different. Guangdong Hospital of traditional Chinese medicine has treated SARS patients. Some of them are cured quickly, but they only take a little Chinese medicine without spending too much; some use a lot of hormones, although they have saved their lives, their lung function has been damaged with sequelae; some are even more unfortunate and life-threatening. The prognosis is different. Although the doctor's treatment plays a certain role, but the therapeutic effect is played through the constitution. For those who died, it cannot be said that doctors did not try their best to rescue them. But why are some people saved alive, while others are dead? This is because medication is

only a stage, while constitution determines the process and prognosis of the disease. An expert once said, "a doctor can cure a disease but not his life." That is to say, a doctor can cure a disease, but if the patient's constitution is poor, the doctor's ability cannot be improved. Whether the doctor's treatment plan can play a role depends on whether the patient's physical fitness can be accepted.

In a word, constitution is not an abstract concept, nor can it be summarized by simple good and bad.

5.4 Understanding of constitution and temperament in TCM

There is a detailed description of constitution in *The Inner Canon of the Yellow Emperor* and ancient Chinese medicine literature, which was discovered by the ancients in practice. They found that the formation of constitution was related to congenital factors more than 2500 years ago. "The birth of a man is based on his mother and his father." How do we come from? It is the combination of the two essence of our parents, called Yin essence and Yang essence in traditional Chinese medicine, or the combination of male essence and female blood to form a new life body embryo. Traditional Chinese medicine doesn't talk about embryo, but it has been realized that human is the product of the combination of parents' essence and essence. *The Divine Pivot · Shouyao's Hardness and Softness* records: "human beings are born with hardness and softness, weak and strong, short and long, yin and Yang." We are talking about the problem of constitution. After we are born, there is hardness and softness, and hardness and softness reflect psychological temperament. This is the concept of temperament. Weak and strong is the reaction to the outside world, a problem of resistance. Short and long is a problem of shape and structure; Yin and Yang is the general principle of analyzing things. We look at the ancients from today's perspective. Although they did not put forward such terms as temperament and constitution, they made it very clear that psychological temperament, resistance and morphological structure were actually discussed. According to our definition of temperament and constitution, we are talking about these three parts.

(1) Congenital factors of constitution

For the congenital factors of constitution, *The Inner Canon of the Yellow Emperor* did not elaborate. Modern molecular genetics has shown that parents pass DNA (deoxyribonucleic acid) to their children through germ cells. DNA with a certain structure produces a certain structure of protein. Protein is the basic material of our life. The smaller structure than protein is ribonucleic acid. Proteins with a certain structure bring certain morphological structure and physiological characteristics. So how is our constitution formed? Its material basis is protein, namely ribonucleic acid – DNA.

DNA has a unique double helix ladder structure, and has a unique biosynthesis mode, namely replication. In the process of DNA replication, the genetic information and codes are transcribed and translated into RNA, and then RNA controls the synthesis of various proteins. Because the DNA passed on to you by your parents is not the same as the genetic information and code carried by others, so the physiological structure and physiological function inherited from your parents are different, and your constitution is also different. The role of genes is to expressed in a specific shape through a series of complex biochemical processes, which is the basis of constitution and genetics.

Why it is said that no two leaves in the world are exactly the same, or that everyone's constitution is different in the world? Because there are four nucleotides in DNA, there are endless arrangements in DNA molecules containing millions of base pairs. No two organisms in the world have the same sequence of bases in their DNA, so no two people in the world have the same genetic constitution. According to a hair unearthed from Ma Wang Dui, we can judge whether the tomb is a man or a woman, and what kind of family. This is confirmed by DNA identification. Paternity testing actually measures DNA. Although the DNA of each person is different, people in the same family are similar.

What is the problem of constitution? I think it's about genes. Genes control life traits, growth, reproduction, birth and death, and pass on genetic information to the next generation. The birth and death of a person, how he or she is in this lifetime, and the process of growing strong and aging, etc., are determined at birth. This is the proposition I just said: physical fitness is more determined by congenital genetic factors, and it is difficult for acquired factors to change the influence of congenital factors. Therefore, the problem of constitution is the gene problem mentioned in western medicine, which is why I choose this topic. In fact, the issue of physical fitness is very cutting-edge and very realistic. Many of its mysteries have not been fully clarified.

(2) ACQUIRED FACTORS OF CONSTITUTION

The acquired factor of constitution is age. The so-called age is related to the process of growth and development. In the book of *Plain Questions Ancient Innocence*, people are divided into: growth and development period (women 7–14 years old, men 8–16 years old), in which kidney qi gradually flourishes, vigorous period, in which kidney qi is full and stable, aging period, in which kidney qi gradually declines. This shows that the rise and fall of kidney qi is the material basis for the process of growth, growth, strength, aging and decline. Therefore, why do we have to take tonifying drugs to fight aging? That's what it means.

All the so-called drugs for immortality found by emperors in the past dynasties are actually kidney tonics. Although there is no medicine for immortality in the world, the theory of Inner Canon of the Yellow Emperor has a great influence on Chinese people. Why is Cordyceps very expensive, because it is tonifying the kidney, can delay aging. Although aging is irresistible, the process can be delayed. Inner Canon of the Yellow Emperor tells us that the rise and fall of kidney qi determines the rise and fall of your constitution. Congenital factors cannot be changed, but acquired factors can. Cordyceps sinensis can improve physical fitness, in line with the concept of traditional Chinese medicine.

From the point of age, we'll talk about both the young and the elderly:

1) Children's Constitution

What are the physical characteristics of children? In the book *Pediatrics Play*, it mentioned that children's "liver often surplus, spleen often insufficient." Let me give an example. When a child has a fever up to 39°C, he will have cramps. Because the liver is often surplus in children, the liver dominates the wind. Once there is a fever, the liver wind moves inward, so it will be cramped. Adults seldom have cramps, and cramps will occur only at 42°C. Some children's nervous system development is not perfect, if the body temperature reaches 38.5°C, they will have cramps. This is the manifestation of "liver often has surplus," which is summarized by the ancients through long-term observation.

How is "Spleen often insufficient"? Because the spleen and the stomach help people digest nutrients, so pediatrics to see spleen and stomach disease in particular. Children are easy to have stomach problems, or not willing to eat, or eat indiscriminately, so it is easy to have spleen and stomach problems. But children's digestive disease is easy to be cured, unlike adult spleen and stomach disease, it seems more difficult, because children are pure Yang body.

It is mentioned in *Children's Medicine Syndrome* that "the five viscera and six Fu organs of children are not complete or complete but not strong." That is to say, children have five internal organs, but they are not mature enough, not strong enough, relatively poor resistance, weak viscera, easy to empty, easy to solid, easy to get cold and hot. "Yi" means that the change is very fast. The fever may reach 38°C and 39°C after half an hour after getting cold, or it may drop to 36°C after a short time when it has just reached 39°C or 40°C. Therefore, children's diseases are easy to change. Some children are still rescuing in the morning and clamoring to eat in the afternoon. They get sick quickly and get better soon. This is the children's constitution "weak viscera, easy to empty, easy to solid, easy to cold and easy to heat." Among the 13 branches of traditional Chinese medicine, pediatrics is the most difficult. Because pediatrics is a department of dumb, only relying on parents, children only know how to cry. Young parents may have to have five or six children before they have any experience. Otherwise, they can't understand whether the child has a stomachache or a sore throat, a secret stool or a fever and headache. There is also a child's disease is easy to change, more difficult to treat. Behind these words is actually about physical problems. When the child is 15 or 16 years old, all aspects of the nervous system are mature and stable, and their constitution will not reach a relatively stable state. Instability and variety are the characteristics of children's constitution.

2) Constitution of the elderly

The physical characteristics of the elderly are "kidney is often insufficient": after 40 years old, Yin Qi gradually weakens and Yin essence in kidney is deficient. Old people often lack of kidney, which leads to the decline in sexual function, nocturnal urine, suffering from prostatitis. Some old women are easy to suffer from chronic cystitis. After cystitis is cured, it is easy for them to urinate on their pants as soon as they cough. Because the kidney dominates the bladder, the kidney division two stools, the manifestation for kidney deficiency cannot be solid, urination cannot help, serious patients often have urinary incontinence.

Old people often have excess liver. Old people get hypertension more, kidney deficiency liver is prosperous, liver prosperous will lead to dizzy. Western Medicine said that cerebral atherosclerosis, our Chinese medicine called liver yang hyperactivity, blood pressure increased. Elderly people are also prone to senile primary tremor, Parkinson's disease, which is "kidney often insufficient, liver often surplus" manifestation. "Kidney often insufficient" manifestation for kidney deficiency, "liver often surplus" for vertigo, convulsion, tremor, faltering.

In addition, "old people have more blood stasis." The human body is made up of Qi and blood. Why do you look ruddy when you are young, walk briskly, and your brain reacts well, because Qi and blood are very vigorous; when you are old, your blood flow is slow due to deficiency of Qi and blood. There are two reasons for aging, one is atherosclerosis; the other is tissue blood supply deficiency, which indicates that the function begins to decline. For example: the lack of blood supply to the heart, manifested as myocardial ischemia, chest tightness, palpitation, insomnia, night sweats, etc.; insufficient blood supply to the brain, manifested as dizziness, dizziness, memory loss, work efficiency is not very high, listening to class is not concentrated; lung blood supply is manifested as asthma, pale face, easy to catch a cold, climbing stairs, heart rate is very fast. Blood stasis is the manifestation of disorder of Qi and blood. Cardiovascular disease are the primary causes of aging and death. Aging begins with blood vessels, indicating that there is blood stasis in the blood vessels. Western Medicine says that there are plaques inside, which Chinese medicines called blood stasis. With plaques, it is obvious that the blood vessels are blocked. If the blood vessels are blocked, the function of the tissues will decline, and the function will decline step by step. If the blood supply becomes more and more insufficient, and finally the blood vessels are blocked, people will die suddenly. This is the characteristic of old people's constitution.

Therefore, the elderly should not only take drugs for tonifying liver and kidney, but also drugs for promoting blood circulation and removing blood stasis, because "the elderly have more blood stasis." Now some old people take some Panax Notoginseng Powder under the guidance of doctors and drink saffron tea to prevent blood stasis, plaque and blood vessel blockage. Once the cardiovascular block, mild angina pectoris, severe myocardial infarction. If the cerebral blood vessels are blocked, the cerebral infarction will occur, and the mild degree may be rescued, but the sequelae may be hemiplegia; the severe may not wake up, because the degree of blood stasis is not the same.

(3) Sex factor of constitution

The female of 17–27 years old and the male of 18–28 years old grow gradually. Girls have menstruation from 13 to 14 years old, and boys have ejaculation from 16 to 18 years old, which indicates that sexual function is mature. The time difference between men and women is 1–2 years old. Girls develop early, boys develop slowly. This is because the difference of chromosome between men and women determines the difference of their constitution.

For example, it is mentioned in "*Divine Pivot · Five Tones and Five Flavors*" that "the birth of a woman has more Qi but less blood." It's easy for women to get angry. Zhu Danxi said that the excess of Qi is fire. After the anger was born, he became angry with fire. In traditional Chinese medicine, liver depression turned into fire. Therefore, Qi and blood should be balanced. If there is an excess, it is easy to get angry and easy to stagnate. "More Qi bur less blood" is mainly manifested in two turning points: one is the growth and development period, the other is menopause. Why thy don't have enough blood? Because women's menstruation, belt, fetus and childbirth all need to lose blood, so it's right to take a little blood tonic medicine, which is based on *The Inner Canon of the Yellow Emperor*. As long as you need it, men can eat donkey hide gelatin. Men also have blood deficiency, but women have more blood deficiency, which reflects a physical tendency.

"*Gynecological Jade Ruler*" mentioned that "women to blood, men to essence." Later generations also have a saying that "women are born with the liver, and men are born with the kidney." Why? This involves the theory of traditional Chinese medicine, that is, liver stores blood and kidney stores essence. Men always have kidney deficiency. Men should tonify kidney and women should replenish blood. Physical problems are behind these facts.

Women are born with the liver. What is the function of liver? At the same time, the liver stores blood, Qi and blood are related to the liver. Therefore, women's "liver is congenital," women's menstruation, belt, fetus, birth defects will cause liver qi stagnation, qi stagnation and blood stasis.

(4) Environmental factors of constitution

According to ecology, all the chemical substances existing in organisms come from soil, air and water. Because the chemical compositions in the crust of different regions are different, the water quality and plant composition are also different, and the constitution of animals and people is also different. For people's constitution, what comes from nature is given by parents, and there is no way to change it. The day after tomorrow is related to environmental factors. There is a saying that "one side of soil and water nurtures one side of people." Shanghainese eat plants grown in the soil of Shanghai, breathe the air of Shanghai, and drink the water of Huangpu River to grow up. There are some unique trace elements, minerals and other substances in the soil, air and water, so one side of the soil and water creates the other side's constitution.

Why are Harbin people and Shandong people tall and big? Because the soil and water over there has raised their tall and big race. Why are Zhejiang people, Guangxi people and Shanghai people relatively short? Because the geographical conditions of life are different, the eating habits are also different.

Congenital factors are given by parents, we have no choice; but acquired factors affect the evolution of constitution to a certain extent. Some people say that I was always sick when I was a child, and then I would not get sick when I was strong. This shows that my constitution is not unchangeable. Personal overall physical fitness is determined by parents, but the acquired environmental factors are related to your height and physical strength. Now our conditions are good, we eat very well, social medical conditions are very good, relatively speaking, it is conducive to the formation of a good constitution.

(5) Classification of temperament and constitution

1) Classification of temperament and constitution in Western Medicine
Hippocrates, the father of Western medicine, believes that human beings are made

up of four kinds of liquids. Different liquids make different temperament, and there are predictive elements in it. Many concepts in *The Inner Canon of the Yellow Emperor* come from practice and speculation. The expression of temperament described by Hippocrates is the special state of mind that I have just mentioned. These four qualities are as follows:

(1) Choleric temperament: Bold, bold and aggressive.

(2) Sanguineness temperament: agile, optimistic, frivolous and changeable.

(3) Mucus temperament: calm, relaxed, weak, able to distinguish right from wrong.

(4) Depressive temperament: thinking much, doubting heavily, imagining wildly, pessimism and disappointment, cowardice.

2) TCM classification of temperament and constitution

Constitution of Traditional Chinese Medicine is divided into nine types:

(1) Peaceful temperament (normal quality): the personality is more open and easy-going, physiological, psychological, morphological aspects are very normal, ancient called peaceful quality, also known as normal quality.

(2) Temperament of Qi deficiency: a person is always lack of strength, which is often seen in life. Some people have food and clothing, and sleep well, but they always have no strength. It seems that they have no strength all their life. In fact, it is because of their Qi deficiency constitution, which may be congenital deficiency, or they may lose their nourishment the day after tomorrow. People with Qi deficiency are easy to catch cold, asthma and respiratory diseases; they are also prone to spontaneous sweating and night sweats. If they move a little, they will be panting and sweating.

(3) Temperament of Yang deficiency: many girls see a doctor, there is no discomfort, is particularly afraid of the cold in winter, hands and feet are cold. Is this sick? No disease, Yang deficiency quality of people is cold hands and feet, clothes wear particularly much, and the susceptibility to cold is strong. If the weather is a little bit cold, they will get sick, but they are not afraid of the heat. If you turn on the air conditioner in summer, they will be too cold to bear. There are also some climacteric female comrades who are hot and cold at one time, which is also Yang deficiency constitution. When this kind of person infects pneumonia, the body temperature often won't rise very high, usually manifestation is medium fever, and easy to become toxic pneumonia. General symptoms of pneumonia are high fever, cough, expectoration, chest pain. But people with Yang deficiency constitution only have a little cough when they get pneumonia. Their body temperature is $37.5\,^{\circ}$C. The fever can not come out and the energy of Yang deficiency is insufficient.

(4) Temperament of Yin deficiency: people with Yin deficiency constitution always have hot palms, dry mouth and dry tongue, their tongue is always red, and

their stools are often secret. Even if it is cold outside, the skin is still hot. This kind of person is easier to get diabetes, yin deficiency and internal heat, and is thinner. As Zhu Danxi said, "thin people have more fire."

(5) Temperament of Phlegm dampness: Zhu Danxi said, "fat people are wet." Phlegm dampness of the people are usually fat, especially weak, a cold, a check of high blood fat, high blood pressure, bleb swelling, metabolic dysfunction. The specific manifestations are metabolic syndrome, obesity, hyperlipidemia, hypertension, hyperglycemia, or the three high are at the critical point. It is called X syndrome, metabolic syndrome and insulin resistance syndrome. People with phlegm dampness constitution are most likely to have cardiovascular and cerebrovascular diseases.

(6) Temperament of Dampness and heat: the important feature of this constitution is that the tongue coating is always yellow and greasy, and the Chinese medicine can not be changed. Hyperlipidemia may often occur. The urine is often yellow, and the stool is secret. The appetite is poor. The chest is stuffy and tired.

(7) Temperament of Blood stasis: this kind of person is born with high blood viscosity, and several blood viscosity indexes of Hemorheology examination are on the high side. When having a physical examination, he should check his blood viscosity (Hemorheology). People with blood stasis constitution tend to have platelet aggregation, high blood viscosity, easy to form plaques, cardiovascular and cerebrovascular diseases, myocardial infarction, cerebral infarction, tissue blood supply insufficiency and other vascular diseases. Some people's tongue is often dark purple, the sublingual vein is swollen and blue purple, which shows blood stasis. If possible, people over 40 or 50 years old can check the carotid artery B ultrasound, coronary artery CT, abdominal aorta B ultrasound, lower extremity artery and vein B ultrasound to see if there are plaques.

(8) Temperament of Qi stagnation: equivalent to Hippocratic depression. People with this temperament are easy to get angry. If you ask him how he sleeps, he may say he can sleep if he has nothing to do, but can't sleep if he has something to do. I asked him what was the matter, and he said I didn't know. In fact, he was well fed and clothed, but he couldn't be happy. He was always depressed and sentimental, and thought of everything in a bad way. This kind of person is most likely to suffer from autism, and then further develop into anxiety disorder or autism, and anxiety disorder alternates.

(9) Temperament of Special quality: allergic constitution. There are so many people like this. Now children are flowers and plants in the greenhouse. In the past, parents gave birth to five or six children, and they were all fine. Now, children are weaker. They are allergic to pollen, banana and oil smoke. Therefore, they are easy to get many skin diseases, asthma, chronic rhinitis and chronic pharyngitis. There are

many unexplained allergic phenomena. Sometimes, they can't find the allergen. They are allergic to eating hairtail seafood, cotton blanket dust, and inhalable particles Substance (PM2.5) allergy, as if anything will cause allergy.

(6) Constitution and health

1) Constitution and disease occurrence
Physical strength is closely related to the disease. Whether the external lethal factors can invade into the human body and whether the individual is sick or not depends largely on the individual's constitution. People with strong resistance do not get sick, while those with weak resistance will get sick.

2) Constitution and tendency of disease
Due to the specificity of individual constitution, individuals are susceptible to some pathogenic factors, or to some diseases. Why? For example, today is extremely cold, some people always catch cold; some people suffer from asthma as soon as they are cold, which is a disease of respiratory system; some people have diarrhea or stomachache or diarrhea as soon as they are cold; some people have joint pain when they are cold, which is manifested as rheumatism and rheumatoid diseases. This is the tendency of the disease, which is determined by the constitution. Therefore, constitution determines the tendency and susceptibility of the disease.

Everyone is faced with a variety of external stimuli. According to the western medicine, it can be summarized as the pathogenic factors of microorganism, physics and chemistry, and those pathogenic factors are always present. Heaven is very fair, social environment and natural environment both will act on people. This person is not abstract, but a person with a physical tendency. A special constitution is susceptible to certain pathogenic factors, which is called "sensation and response" in traditional Chinese medicine. As I said just now, there are people who are particularly sensitive to the cold virus, especially to the cold. Some people are not adapted to the heat. When it's 38°C outside in summer, he will have a poor appetite, feel limb fatigue and get sweating. In fact, there is no disease, but the fact that this constitution does not adapt to the summer heat.

Pathogenic factors react to people. Western medicine has defined this as a reaction to external environmental stimuli. External environmental stimulation includes biological, physical and chemical, as well as wind, cold, heat, dampness, dry, fire, joy, anger, worry, sadness and panic, etc. this reaction works through constitution, that is, the reaction produced by pathogenic factors acting on people's constitution is manifested as disease. People have a physical tendency, which is different by person.

This process is called qualitative, which is the change process from constitution to transformation. TCM syndrome differentiation mainly distinguishes two aspects, one is to distinguish the constitution, the other is to distinguish the clinical manifestations, these two aspects together come to the syndrome of TCM. Western medicine stresses disease and syndrome. No matter the syndrome or the disease or the syndrome is, they all belong to the result of the comprehensive reaction of the human or the constitution to the pathogenic factors, which is manifested as various clinical symptoms. If you understand this, you can understand how the disease is formed and why different constitutions have different manifestations? Because physical fitness acts as a lever.

3) The principle behind "different treatment for the same disease, same treatment for different diseases" in TCM
The underlying principle of "different treatment for the same disease" is: the etiology is the same, but the manifestation is different due to different constitution, so the same disease is treated differently. "Treating different diseases at the same time" means although they are different diseases, but the principle of treatment is the same. The underlying principle is: Although the etiology is different, but the constitution of patients is the same, the disease and syndrome are the same, so different diseases are treated at the same time. Why under the same pneumonia, you take this medicine and you feel good, while he is not, or his disease get even more and more serious? This is because "the etiology is the same, the constitution is different," so the result and prognosis are not the same.

In terms of treatment, western medicine treats from the cause of disease, while traditional Chinese medicine focuses on the regulation of constitution. This is the difference between western medicine and traditional Chinese medicine. Constitution affects the formation of disease syndrome, and restricts the transmission and transformation of disease syndrome. The process of disease in everyone is always the function of constitution.

Once diagnosed as pneumonia by western medicine, the treatment plan is the same; for SARS, the treatment plan is the same; for malignant tumor, the treatment strategy is the same. But traditional Chinese medicine is not the same, because each person's constitution is not the same, the disease manifestation is not the same, even if the same disease treatment plan is not the same. Traditional Chinese medicine should be based on individual conditions, and it should be based on the constitution.

It emphasizes that "If it is urgent, it should be treated with its treetop; if it slows down, it should be treated at its root." From the point of constitution, "if you are urgent, you should treat your symptoms; if you slow down, you should treat your constitution." For example, when facing an emergency coma patient, of course, you must try to rescue first. When facing a patient with a high fever, of course, you must first release him from this fever. And when facing a patient who is extremely painful, first of all, you must let him not feel pain, which is called "palliative treatment." When the fever subsides and the pain subsides, it is necessary to "treat the root of the disease if it slows down." This "root" is to strengthen the body, that is, to improve his constitution. For example, if a patient comes to see a headache, he should first let him not hurt, and then let him come to you next time. What's your second visit? To prevent him from having a headache again. Then the doctor should "strengthen the body," which is to improve his constitution. A patient with cancer has been treated with western surgery, radiotherapy and chemotherapy, and is basically stable. Let's look at traditional Chinese medicine, that is, strengthening the body and improving the constitution. The first is to improve his immune capacity to prevent recurrence and metastasis; the second is to improve his symptoms and improve the quality of life. These are the two principles of TCM treatment.

A large number of clinical practices of traditional Chinese medicine has proved that different constitutions cause different response to treatment by the same method. Therefore, TCM pays attention to syndrome differentiation. Western medicine is said to be drug compliance, the constitution of how to adapt to drugs, adaptation will have effect. No adaption, no effect. And even produce adverse reactions, which causes liver damage. Therefore, many problems and phenomena can be easily solved from the perspective of constitution.

4) The significance of studying constitution
(1) The concept of TCM constitution theory is the unity of form and spirit, which combines human structure and function, constitution and temperament. This research method from the overall perspective of the unity of form and spirit is a new perspective, which can promote the development of medicine.

(2) Academician Wu Jieping once said: "medicine in the 21st century is individualized treatment. The theoretical basis of individualized treatment is the theory of constitution. If we grasp the theory of constitution, we can realize individualized treatment." US President Barack Obama proposed precision medicine, which is to understand the mechanism of disease formation by analyzing the genetic information, environmental factors and lifestyle of the population, and then develop corresponding drugs to implement individualized precision treatment. That is to say, check the gene of the person before treatment. He must be sick because of gene problems, especially those diseases that cannot be cured, such as cancer, hypertension, cardiovascular disease, etc., are all gene problems. Precise treatment is to change the patient's genes on the basis of understanding the genes. Precise therapy is gene therapy, the premise is to understand genes. The principle of traditional Chinese

medicine is to understand the patient's constitution. This two look different, but the basic principle is the same.

The essence of traditional Chinese medicine (TCM) is to emphasize the essence of TCM precise treatment.

LECTURE 6

Differentiation of Personality and Body Constitution

Body-mind Regulation of Five-Status

LECTURER: YANG QIULI

Introduction to the speaker:

Yang Qiuli is a scientist and a supervisor for postgraduate students in Chinese Academy of Chinese Medical Sciences. She graduated from Beijing University of Chinese Medicine in July 1984. She commits herself to research, clinical practice and teaching of TCM psychology, personality, body constitution and mental health, psychosomatic health, health preservation, etc. She is one of the founders of the first indigenous measure of personality assessment of Five-Status Personality Test and Five-Five Body Constitution Test in China. Body-mind Regulation System of Five-Status is the standardized measure of mental and physical health assessment in TCM.

hinese culture in the past thousands of years, as well as *The Inner Canon of the Yellow Emperor* (*Huáng Dì Nèi Jīng*, 黄帝内经), laid a solid foundation for the development of TCM psychology. We try to create psychosomatic testing, involving both mental and physical health assessments. That embodies the concept of "intact body-mind" in traditional Chinese medicine, putting emphasize on psychosomatic medicine for health care.

Personalities and body constitutions are closely related in TCM, which is the embodiment of holism. Only when people are healthy both physically and mentally can they be regarded as enjoying good health. In *The Inner Canon of the Yellow Emperor* (*Huáng Dì Nèi Jīng*, 黄帝内经), there are "five-status classification" based on Yin-Yang theory and "five-element classification" based on five-element theory, to categorize people based on personalities and body constitutions. Personalities and body constitutions begin before birth, which are also influenced by environment after birth involving life, work and school. Body-mind harmony is the key to stay healthy physically and mentally.

This lecture mainly introduces two standardized assessment tools of "Five-Status Personality Test" and "Five-Five Body Constitution Test." They are commonly used in TCM to classify personalities and body constitutions, assessing overall health. The "Five-Status Personality Test" can be used to reveal psychological states, while "Five-Five Body Constitution Test" can be used to determine physiological states. "Body-mind Regulation System of Five-Status" is established to provide personalized plans for health regulation involving psychotherapy, diet therapy, sports, music, physiotherapy, medicated diet and so on, based on test results as well as TCM theories and clinical experience of health preservation. Nowadays, it is of great significance to provide individualized plans for overall health regulation based on test results and clinical experience, considering the national strategy to develop a "Healthy China" and demands expressed by citizens in China. In addition, the test results can not only help to assess mental and physical health for health preservation, but also be used as evidence for diagnosing mental illness and psychosomatic disorders.

The body in the "intact body-mind" includes both external physiques and internal physiological functions. Body Constitution Test is used to assess internal physiological functions. The mind in the "intact body-mind" refers to mental health, revealing psychological state. "The body contains the mind, while the mind dominates the body." That is to say, the mind can control the body, and the mind exists based on the body. The expression of "intact body-mind" concisely describes human life.

6.1 Health – the eternal theme of building a harmonious society

Life is the most precious to people, and health is the greatest wealth. Health is the basic condition for human beings to contribute to society, an important prerequisite for the prosperity of a nation, and a significant foundation for building a civilized and harmonious society. In 1989, the World Health Organization of the United Nations put forward that health was a state of complete physical, mental and social well-being and not merely the absence of disease or infirmity. The absence of disease or infirmity is only a basic aspect of health that requires the normal state of body and mind as well as living in harmony with social and natural environments, which is a new concept of holism for health.

Health relies on body constitutions, and body constitutions depend on "mind and body" referring to personalities and types of body constitution. The holistic view of "correspondence between nature and human" and "intact body-mind," involving a space-time biopsychosocial model, is more advanced than the new Western medical model, which has been taken as a clinical practice guideline. TCM always attaches importance to holism, regarding the human body as an organic whole that is integrated with natural and social environments. The harmony between body and mind is the key for health preservation and disease prevention. Personalities and body constitutions can not only demonstrate physical and mental health status, but also act as the basis of disease occurrence. A person with positive character traits, a moderate and healthy body constitution, as well as a healthy lifestyle, is in a normal state of physical and mental health. Based on that, the person, who can restrain and control thinking and actions well according to the morality recognized by society, is in a perfect state of health.

6.2 Medical models and views on health care

Clinical practice is based on medical models. The change of medical models helped people have a more comprehensive understanding of health. In the past, modern medicine emphasized more on the biomedical model. With the development of medicine, Professor Engel put forward the biopsychosocial model in 1979, which pays more attention to the influence of social factors and psychological factors on health. For thousands of years, TCM has paid attention to "correspondence between nature and human" and "intact body-mind." During treatment and diagnosis in TCM, change of seasons, geographical environments, social environments and individual factors, are all taken into consideration. Medical literature of the past dynasties records that TCM always emphasizes the relationship between human and nature and the influence of nature on human beings. Therefore, in 2000, Professor Xue Chongcheng and I put forward the medical model of traditional Chinese medicine, namely the "space-time biopsychosocial model." From this model, we can see what TCM contains. The development of medical models in Western medicine does not change with the development of medicine, which are improved based on clinical experience. The space-time biopsychosocial model in TCM is advanced and forward-looking, which began when *The Inner Canon of the Yellow Emperor* (*Huáng Dì Nèi Jīng*, 黄帝内经) was completed. It attaches importance to the influence of social factors, natural environments and personal psychological factors on health, which brings TCM advantages compared with western medicine or traditional medicine in other countries.

6.3 Understanding of health

Nowadays, the spectrum of disease has changed, with increasing chronic diseases and psychosomatic diseases and mental illness. Psychological factors are very important to health. In 1989, the World Health Organization put forward that health was a state of complete physical, mental and social well-being and not merely the absence of disease or infirmity. Therefore, doctors should pay attention to the mental health of patients in clinical practice, and identify whether they are in the normal state of overall health according to the morality and ethics recognized by society.

How can we understand health? To evaluate the state of health requires an overall assessment of mind and body. A healthy person is mentally energetic, optimistic, and positive, who is able to solve problems and adapt to social environments. Mental health is influenced by individual and social factors. According to the World Health Organization, health involves immunity to the common cold and resistance to general infections, as well as the overall state of proper body weight, balanced physique, good sleep, coordinated movements, shiny hair, bright eyes, etc.

6.4 Understanding of health in TCM

Although there is no clear definition of health in TCM, healthy conditions are summarized as "correspondence between nature and human," "intact body-mind" and "balanced yin and yang," containing broad connotations. TCM believes that Qi and blood are the most basic motive force and substance of life. Therefore, the coordinated operation of Qi and blood in the body is the most basic guarantee for people to keep healthy. Only in this way can mind and body maintain a relatively balanced and healthy state. Therefore, the harmony between Qi and blood is critical to the harmony between mind and body, which must be achieved to successfully adapt to natural environments in a healthy state. Those are based on my views put forward 10 years ago, which refer to "harmony between Qi and blood," "harmony between body and mind" and "harmony between nature and human" (as shown in Figure 6-1). The article was published in *Chinese Journal of Basic Medicine in Traditional Chinese Medicine* in February 2011. They are consistent with the WHO's definition of health. Health in TCM involves the relationship between human and nature, with richer connotations.

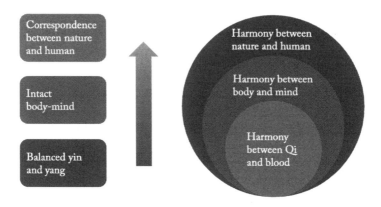

Figure 6-1   Understanding of health in TCM

6.5   Factors affecting health

Based on TCM etiology, the factors affecting health can be divided into three categories: internal factors, external factors, and factors neither internal nor external.

(1) Internal factors: individual personality traits and body constitutions (different types of body constitution).

(2) External factors: natural and social environments. Natural environments include the change in nature, involving air, water, soil, and geography. Social environments are the places where we live and work, including the surrounding interpersonal relationships and healthcare systems.

(3) Factors neither internal nor external: lifestyles. It includes clothing, food, housing, transportation, work, entertainment, social interaction, manners, etc. Values, morality and aesthetics are closely related to personality traits, which affect lifestyles. Many diseases (including tumors) are caused by bad lifestyles. Lifestyles are influenced not only by personality traits, but also by working and living conditions. There are

so many factors affecting lifestyles, which further affect physical and mental health. Nowadays, many chronic diseases are caused by bad lifestyles.

Actually, external causes work internally. Any external factors that affect health have impact on the body internally.

Some people are outgoing but some are introverted. Some people are friendly but some are selfish. Why is it so? Some people have anxiety, tension, and depression, but some people are calm in the face of pressure. Some people are full of energy with ruddy cheeks, but some people get irritable with insomnia after eating Renshen (人 参, Radix Ginseng) and Lurong (鹿茸, Cornu Cervi Pantotrichum). Some people catch colds, but some do not when the weather changes. Different people can have different symptoms after catching colds. Those phenomena are closely related to personality traits and body constitutions.

The changes of weather can have impacts on persons with Yang deficiency and Qi deficiency, who have weakened immune systems. If they pay attention to health preservation, dressing properly, sticking to healthy diets, and good lifestyles, they may not be attacked by the external pathological factors of wind-cold. But if they are not aware of Yang Qi deficiency and doesn't care about the change of weather, they may have colds and other diseases. Therefore, the external factors of change in weather take effects based on individual internal conditions. People with good personality traits and healthy mental states can often actively face problems, pressures and disasters, as well as successfully adapt to social environments, which are significant for the prevention of psychological and psychosomatic disorders.

In addition to good personality traits, people need proper body constitutions to stay healthy. Bad lifestyles can break the balance between yin and yang. Mild imbalance leads to sub-health state, while serious imbalance causes diseases. Preventive treatment is to maintain and improve health on the one hand and is to restore health on the other hand with diets, sports and medications when sub-health occurs, rebalancing yin and yang. Those states can be assessed by tests. Good personality traits and body constitutions are key to maintain mental and physical health.

Today, about 70% of the whole population are in sub-health condition, according to the World Health Organization. 25% of the population have diseases, and only 5% are relatively healthy. It can be seen that most people are in sub-health condition. People with sub-health can have body constitutions of imbalance and negative personality traits. 70% of the people with diseases have psychosomatic disorders, caused by psychosocial factors, implying the importance of mental health. Most of the psychosomatic disorders are caused by bad lifestyles, including hypertension, coronary heart disease, tumors, obesity, cerebrovascular disease, cardiovascular disease, implying the significance of good lifestyles.

Personalities and body constitutions are internal factors affecting health, while lifestyles are factors neither internal nor external. Although we cannot choose innate qualities, we can improve personalities and body constitutions through cultivating good habits. Personalities and body constitutions are relatively stable, but they can change by time. In order to maintain good health, it is very important to understand what personality traits and which body constitution you have. Then you can regulate physical can mental health accordingly and properly.

6.6   Understanding of personalities and body constitutions

How do we get to know ourselves? Tests can help. In clinic, B-ultrasound, X-ray, CT scan and MRI can be used to diagnose diseases. But they cannot be used for sub-health involving depression, anxiety, tension, these problems, for which scales can help. Different people have different personality traits and body constitutions, thus making everyone unique.

In modern psychology, there are many personality scales, including EPQ, MMPI and 16PF. According to the five-status classification in *The Inner Canon of the Yellow Emperor* (*Huáng Dì Nèi Jīng*, 黄帝内经) · *Correspondence between Man and Nature*, we created "Five-Status Personality Test," the first indigenous measure of personality assessment in China, based on modern methods of psychological scale construction. Through standardization, we achieved test norms in different aspects, nationally and regionally. In clinical practice, the mental health assessment test includes different scales for depression, anxiety, etc., which helps better understand mental illness.

6.7   Psychological diagnosis and assessment in TCM

(1) Observation, listening and smelling, inquiring, pulse feeling and palpation. TCM assesses mental health and diagnoses psychological disorders through the four techniques of observation, listening and smelling, inquiring, pulse feeling and palpation. When patients enter the consulting room, doctors would look at patients and have general impressions of them, about their facial expressions, skin complexions, postures, behaviors and so on. Listening and smelling is to identify if the speaking voice is low or high and if there is any body odor. Inquiring is to collect information about personalities and body constitutions based on the tests. Pulse feeling and palpation is to examine other aspects of the body. It is of great significance for doctors to understand the overall conditions of disease through the four techniques. Besides, it is also necessary to understand psychological states

and personality traits of patients by means of modern psychological testing for psychological diagnosis.

(2) Treatment based on five-status. During receiving acupuncture and moxibustion, people can experience special sensory conduction along meridians. Those with body constitutions characterized by Yang property would have more intense feelings of sensory conduction along meridians. *The Inner Canon of the Yellow Emperor* (*Huáng Dì Nèi Jīng*, 黄帝内经) reads "ancient doctors good at practicing acupuncture and moxibustion were able to treat patients according to five-status." That implies acupuncturists in ancient times noticed the close relationship between human temperaments and therapeutic effects. Therefore, the temperament of patients should be identified before treatment, and then treatment plans can be made accordingly based on personality traits and body constitutions (five-status), which takes both mental health and physical health into consideration. Proper manipulations of acupuncture and moxibustion can be chosen based on types of nerves and temperaments to improve curative effects in terms of modern medicine. Therefore, treatment based on five-status is to understand personalities of patients, and then to develop comprehensive treatment plans according to specific conditions.

(3) Collecting the information about living habits. *The Inner Canon of the Yellow Emperor* (*Huáng Dì Nèi Jīng*, 黄帝内经) · *Instructions of The Teacher* reads "when people want to enter into another country, they have to get familiar with the customs followed by people in that country; when people want to go to others' family, they must try to know the taboos held in that family; when people want to enter into a hall, they have to inquire about the etiquettes; when doctors treat patients, they must be clear about the preference of patients." Doctors asking about living habits actually show concern for patients. Information such as living habits, family backgrounds, personal hobbies, and social status can help doctors develop better treatment plans. This is to say, doctors must know what patients need at first, and then solve their problems.

(4) Taking personal experience into consideration. Personal experience involves social status and interpersonal relationships in the past and in the current. Mental health and physical health are interrelated, both playing important roles in treating psychosomatic disorders. *Basic Questions* (*Sù Wèn*, 素问) · *Major Discussion on the Changes of Qi-Convergence* reads "the so-called Dao (law) is related to the heavens in the upper, the earth in the lower and human beings in the middle and that is why it can last forever; the position of the heavens means the study of astronomy; the position of the earth means the study of geography; the study of the changes of the human body is known as human affairs." That is to say, doctors must have basic ideas about the surroundings of patients. Some people had been very rich, but went bankrupt later. Life experience could bring impacts on such visitors and patients, so

doctors should take that into consideration. The mentioned principles of diagnosis and treatment quoted from *The Inner Canon of the Yellow Emperor* (*Huáng Dì Nèi Jīng*, 黄帝内经) are only a tip of the iceberg in the book. It can be sees that TCM put equal emphasis on mental health and physical health since ancient times.

To sum up, the treatment principles for psychosomatic disorders in *The Inner Canon of the Yellow Emperor* (*Huáng Dì Nèi Jīng*, 黄帝内经) are treatment based on five-status, collecting the information about living habits, and taking personal experience into consideration. Personality traits, body constitutions, environmental factors of nature and society, must be considered during treating mental illness and psychosomatic disorders because they can make big differences to clinical practice. The related article was published in *Chinese Journal of Basic Medicine in Traditional Chinese Medicine* (*January 2010, Vol. 16, Issue 1*).

(5) Judging the inside from observation of the outside. In TCM, it means getting to know the internal essence by looking at external phenomena. The external refers to symptoms, while the internal refers to mental activities. Speech and behavior of patients can help us understand their mental activities, inferring the overall condition from details.

(6) Comparing the normal and the abnormal. Taking the normal range as criteria, abnormal conditions can be detected. Seven emotions leading to internal damage are of abnormal conditions. With different personality traits, people can have various responses to events to different extents. People with a quick temper act fast and get enraged easily, while gentle persons would act in a different way. It is not appropriate to criticize a person according to personalities of others. Therefore, we identify abnormal conditions of individuals based on the normal conditions of themselves.

(7) Test questionnaires. Self-designed questionnaires and standardized rating scales can assist with clinical assessments. Both "Five-Status Personality Test" and "Five-Five Body Constitution Test" involve questionnaires. Typical questions can be asked to assess the exact situations of patients and visitors, which is a commonly used method for psychological diagnosis.

In my opinion, "intact body-mind" is a better expression than "unity of body and mind" to describe health status. "Unity of body and mind" implies a healthy state of balance between human and nature. Both physical and psychological conditions must be taken into consideration in clinical practice, through which causes of disease can be identified based on psychosomatic disorders.

TCM model of diagnosis and treatment puts emphasis on individualization, by assessing and improving mental and physical heath with four diagnostic methods of observation, listening and smelling, inquiring, pulse feeling and palpation as well as treatments based on individuals, geography, climates and diseases. There are "different treatments for the same disease" in TCM, which also highlights individualization. Compared to some modern medical models, TCM takes mental health and physical health as a whole, treating not only diseases but also the overall health conditions, which demonstrates humanistic care in clinical practice.

6.8 Personalities and body constitutions in TCM

67% of the articles in *The Inner Canon of the Yellow Emperor* (*Huáng Dì Nèi Jīng*, 黄帝内经) are involved in psychiatry and psychology. "Five-status classification" and "five-element classification" discussed in *The Inner Canon of the Yellow Emperor* (*Huáng Dì Nèi Jīng*, 黄帝内经) · *Correspondence between Man and Nature* and *The Inner Canon of the Yellow Emperor* (*Huáng Dì Nèi Jīng*, 黄帝内经) · *Twenty-five Types of People Divided According to Yin and Yang* are the oldest records of personalities and body constitutions. Characteristics of human personalities, body constitutions and physiques are described in details, as well as their classification, relationships among each other, associations with seasons and diseases in clinical practice. It covers the basic contents of personalities, body constitutions and physiques in modern psychology, giving definitions of "soul," "psyche," "mind," "thinking," "considering," "intelligence," "emotion" and "will." "Intact body-mind" and "unity of body and mind" are significant ideas in TCM, so both mental and physical health are considered for causes of disease, pathogenesis, diagnosis, treatment, health preservation, etc., based on TCM system of personalities and body constitutions.

(1) FIVE-STATUS CLASSIFICATION

According to *The Inner Canon of the Yellow Emperor* (*Huáng Dì Nèi Jīng*, 黄帝内经). *Correspondence between Man and Nature*, people are divided into five categories based on yin and yang: Greater Yin, Lesser Yin, Greater Yang, Lesser Yang and Balanced Yin-Yang. Among them, Balanced Yin-Yang refers to a group of people with relatively balanced yin and yang. Greater Yang and Lesser Yang contain more yang and less yin, while Greater Yin and Lesser Yin contain more yin and less Yang. According to *The Inner Canon of the Yellow Emperor* (*Huáng Dì Nèi Jīng*, 黄帝内经) · *Twenty-five Types of People Divided According to Yin and Yang*, people are divided into five categories based on properties of wood, fire, earth, metal and water. Each category is further subdivided into five categories. Altogether, there are "twenty-five types of persons."

The five categories of people with Greater Yin, Lesser Yin, Greater Yang, Lesser Yang and Balanced Yin-Yang have different features. People with Greater Yang contain the most Yang and the least Yin, while people with Greater Yin contain the most Yin and the least Yang, and so on and so forth. Their personalities differ in terms of reactions, determination, temperaments, emotions, behaviors, actions, movements, functions of organs inside the body, etc., based on the quantity of yin and Yang. In this case, Yang implies excitation while yin implies inhibition. In clinical practice, different treatment methods should be adopted according to status (personalities and body constitutions), namely, individualized treatment, which is an advantage of TCM.

1) People of Greater Yin. *The Inner Canon of the Yellow Emperor* (*Huáng Dì Nèi Jīng,* 黄帝内经) reads "people of Greater Yin are greedy; they have no social competence; from the outside they appear to be modest but internally they harbor sinister thoughts; they love to take and they hate to give.; their heart is gentle but does not open; they do not concentrate on a task when the time has come, rather they wait for others to move and act themselves only afterwards." "Being greedy" implies being selfish. There is a kind of people who like to get, but are not willing to give. That "from the outside they appear to be modest but internally they harbor sinister thoughts" refers to being careful and introverted in mind, which cannot be seen from behaviors. That "they do not concentrate on a task when the time has come" refers to unwillingness to pursue fashion or keep pace with new trends. That "they wait for others to move and act themselves only afterwards" refers to following others with lack of initiative. People of Greater Yin are introverted, selfish, self-conscious, sensitive and suspicious, who think deeply about problems, usually going for things that generate profits while quitting when there is no benefit.

2) People of Lesser Yin. *The Inner Canon of the Yellow Emperor* (*Huáng Dì Nèi Jīng,* 黄帝内经) reads "people of Lesser Yin are a little greedy, and they have the heart of a robber; when they realize that others have lost something, they always behave as if they themselves had made a gain; they love to harm, and they love to destroy; when they see that someone else has come to honor, contrary to what one might expect they react with rage; they are envious and lack any compassion." Those people are slightly greedy, thoughtful and creative. In addition, that "when they realize that others have lost something, they always behave as if they themselves had made a gain" means schadenfreude. That "they love to harm, and they love to destroy" refers to being jealous and ungrateful.

3) People of Greater Yang. *The Inner Canon of the Yellow Emperor* (*Huáng Dì Nèi Jīng,* 黄帝内经) reads "people of Greater Yang are content with their existence; they love to make big claims but do not have the required competence, and hence these are empty words; their mind reaches the four regions and when they take

something on, and they do not care whether it is right or wrong; they act randomly and only in their self-interest; when their affairs fail, they never feel remorse." That "they love to make big claims but do not have the required competence, and hence these are empty words" means being arrogant and exaggerating the facts. That "their mind reaches the four regions" implies being ambitious. That "when they take something on, and they do not care whether it is right or wrong" refers to doing things regardless of right and wrong. That "they act randomly and only in their self-interest" refers to being self-sufficient with conceit. That "when their affairs fail, they never feel remorse" means they do not regret in the face of failure.

4) People of Lesser Yang. *The Inner Canon of the Yellow Emperor* (*Huáng Dì Nèi Jīng*, 黄帝内经) reads "pople of Lesser Yang pursue their tasks diligently and have great self-respect; even if they are only minor officials, they still consider themselves something special and well suited; they love to have exchanges with others, and they do not devote themselves to their duties internally; when they stand, they tend to direct their face upward; when they walk, they sway back and forth; their two upper arms and their two elbows are pushed backward." People of Lesser Yang often carefully judge before doing things to avoid carelessness, but they are complacent and arrogant. They have good communication skills, but are not good at dealing with daily routine of tasks. They tend to tilt heads up when standing, and swing bodies when walking. In daily life, they often hold hands behind backs and tend to expose elbows.

5) People of Balanced Yin-Yang. *The Inner Canon of the Yellow Emperor* (*Huáng Dì Nèi Jīng*, 黄帝内经) reads "people of Balanced Yin-Yang live in a peaceful and calm environment; nothing makes them worry; nothing causes them to enjoy; they fulfill their tasks and are always friendly; they never enter into a conflict with others; they wait for changes to occur by themselves; they accept praise with modesty; they argue without intending to regulate; that is called highest achievement in regulation; they are complacent and sociable, they are dignified and yet friendly; they are open towards others, and well-behaved; the masses of people call them gentlemen." That is to say, such people are very graceful and dignified. They are not emotional, who are not pleased by external gains or saddened by personal losses. They are calm and peaceful with the strong ability to adjust themselves.

In *The Inner Canon of the Yellow Emperor* (*Huáng Dì Nèi Jīng*, 黄帝内经), behaviors, manners and expressions are described in detail for five-status classification. People of Greater Yin have a lot of yin without yang, while people of Lesser Yin have more yin with less yang. That is to say, people of Greater Yin have the lowest amount of yang, and people of Lesser Yin have more yang and less yin than people of Greater

Yin. People of Greater Yang and people of Lesser Yang have more yang with less yin, but people of Lesser Yang have more yin and less yang than people of Greater Yang. That is all about the proportion of yin to yang.

(2) Five-element classification

Based on the theory of five elements, "five-element classification" divides people into five types: Wood, Fire, Earth, Metal and Water. The five types of people are described in detail in *The Inner Canon of the Yellow Emperor* (*Huáng Dì Nèi Jīng*, 黄帝内经), involving physiques, personalities, appearance, skin colors, walking postures, adaptability to natural environments in the East, West, North, and South, as well as to weathers in spring, summer, autumn and winter.

1) People of Wood. *The Inner Canon of the Yellow Emperor* (*Huáng Dì Nèi Jīng*, 黄帝内经) reads, "people of Wood follow the presetting of the upper jue tone, who resemble the Green Thearchy." That is to say, people of Wood have the voice of jue tone and look like Cang emperor. "Their complexion is greenish; their head is small; their face is long; their shoulders and their back are big; their body stands up straight; hands and feet are small; they love wealth." It implies such people are talented and intelligent, which can be determined by facial complexion, voice, head size and walking postures. That "they tax their heart; they have little physical strength, and they worry much; they work hard at reaching their tasks" means that this kind of people have more mental work because they have more creative ideas, who tend to think more and worry more. "They can tolerate the weather in spring and summer, but cannot tolerate the weather in autumn and winter; so, in autumn and winter they are subject to attack of coolness and coldness and frequently fall ill; they are analogous to the Liver Channel of Foot-Jueyin and have a calm and amiable disposition." It demonstrates the relationship between human and nature that such people usually stay well in spring and summer but easily get sick in autumn and winter.

2) People of Fire. *The Inner Canon of the Yellow Emperor* (*Huáng Dì Nèi Jīng*, 黄帝内经) reads, "people of Fire follow the presetting of the upper zhi tone, who resemble the Red Thearchy." That is to say, people of Fire have reddish complexion. "They have well-developed shoulders, back, buttocks and abdomen; their hands and feet are small; they do not feel secure when walking on the ground." It explains they are impatient but think quickly and walk steadily, who have broad backs, thin faces, small heads, small hands and feet, with shoulders, backs, thighs and abdomens well developed. That "when they walk fast, their shoulders sway and their back is fleshy" means they have strong muscles, who sway when walking.

This kind of people are smart but lack integrity, who don't put emphasis on money. "Hastiness, short life span and susceptibility to sudden death" implies they are prone to sudden death. That "they can tolerate the weather in spring and summer, but cannot tolerate the weather in autumn and winter; they tend to contract diseases in autumn and winter due to attack of pathogenic factors in these two seasons" demonstrates they easily get sick when it is cold.

3) People of Earth. "They follow the presetting of the upper gong tone, who resemble the Yellow Thearchy; they have yellow complexion and round face; their head is big, with handsome shoulders and back, a large abdomen, nice thighs and lower legs, small hands and feet, and much flesh; the upper and the lower are balanced; they walk securely on the ground, and lift their feet only a little; their heart is peaceful; they love to be of use to others, and they find no pleasure in power and violence; they tend to associate with other people; they can tolerate the weather in autumn and winter, but cannot tolerate the weather in spring and summer; when attacked by pathogenic factors in spring and summer, they will fall ill; this type of people are honest and sincere." People of Earth are characterized by yellow skin, round face, big head, well-developed shoulders and back, large abdomen, slender legs, small hands and feet, plump muscles, and well-balanced physique. They are gentle and prudent, walking steadily and quietly, who are willing to help others and good at uniting people, but do not curry favor with authorities. They can tolerate the cold in autumn and winter, but are vulnerable to warm heat in spring and summer.

4) People of Metal. "They follow the presetting of the upper shang tones, who resemble the White Thearchy; they have square face and white complexion; their head is small with small shoulders and back and a little abdomen; their hands and feet are small; heel bones protrude; their skeleton is light; their body is faultless; their heart is tense, calm and adventurous; they are well suited for an official career; they can tolerate the weather in autumn arid winter, but cannot tolerate the weather in spring and summer; when attacked by pathogenic factors in spring and summer, they will fall ill; this type of people are analogous to the Lung Channel of Hand-Taiyin; they are firm and indomitable." Such people are characterized by white skin, square face, small head, thin shoulder and back, small abdomen, small hands and feet, and strong heels. They are brisk, honest and irritable, who keep silent when staying quiet and move fast when taking action. Such people are suitable to work as government officials. They can tolerate the cold in autumn and winter, but are vulnerable to warm heat in spring and summer.

5) People of Water. "They follow the presetting of the upper shang tone, who resemble the Black Thearchy; they are people of black complexion and uneven face; their head is big, and their chin is edged; their shoulders are small with

big abdomen; they move hands and feet; when walking, their body sways; their tailbone is long; their back is extended; they have no respect to and fear of others, frequently cheating and bullying others, and often getting massacred; they can tolerate the weather in autumn and winter, but cannot tolerate the weather in spring and summer; when attacked by pathogenic factors in spring and summer, they will fall ill; this type of people are analogous to the Kidney Channel of Foot-Shaoyin and are base in personality. Such people are characterized by black skin, uneven face, big head, broad cheek, thin shoulders, and big abdomen. They are active, who sway when walking, with long sacra and tailbones as well as long spines. Good at deception, they do not respect or fear anyone, who are prone to murder. They can tolerate the cold in autumn and winter, but are vulnerable to warm heat in spring and summer.

"Five-element classification" is recorded in detail and systematically in *The Inner Canon of the Yellow Emperor* (*Huáng Dì Nèi Jīng*, 黄帝内经), which is similar to the classification system, developed by Kretschmer (1888–1964), that correlates body build and physical constitution with personality characteristics. According to the system based on physique, the five sense organs, skin color, hair, and postures, there are body types including leptosomic, athletic, pyknic, abnormal and mixed, corresponding to Wood, Earth, Fire, Water and Metal. Both systems describe personality traits in similar ways. But Kretschmer's work was published in 1921, two thousand years later than *The Inner Canon of the Yellow Emperor* (*Huáng Dì Nèi Jīng*, 黄帝内经) had come out.

(3) Personality traits based on "five-status classification"

1) People of Greater Yin are modest, suspicious, thoughtful, pessimistic, timid and cowardly, who do not lead but follow. They are feminine, indecisive, introspective, lonely, conservative, and selfish, without interest in excitements or fashions, who do not tend to believe others easily.

2) People of Lesser Yin are calm, thoughtful, good at distinguishing right from wrong, self-disciplined, and jealousy. They are indecisive, cautious and practical, with endurance, who do not speak or act rashly.

3) People of Greater Yang are brave, enterprising, resolute, arrogant, impulsive, and emotional, who dare to insist on their own views, dare to put forward opinions, and are not afraid of failure.

4) People of Lesser Yang are agile, optimistic, sociable, cheerful, capricious, witty, active, easygoing, and casual, who like to talk and laugh, fond of literary and artistic activities, but do not like staying quiet to think deeply.

5) People of Balanced Yin-Yang are very calm, dignified, modest, but not emotional. In addition, they are selfless and fearless, who are not pleased by external gains or saddened by personal losses, so they are able to adjust according to rules of development and keep themselves balanced.

(4) CHARACTERISTICS OF "FIVE-STATUS CLASSIFICATION" AND "FIVE-ELEMENT CLASSIFICATION"

According to the development of modern psychology and *The Inner Canon of the Yellow Emperor* (*Huáng Dì Nèi Jīng*, 黄帝内经), "five-status classification" is more suitable for personality tests, involving emotional experience, cognitive process, willpower, mindset and behavior.

"Five-element classification" is based on appearance, skin color and physique. The physique involves facial complexion, the size of head, shoulder and back, the length of limbs, walking postures, and the adaptability to nature. "Correspondence between nature and human" in TCM is embodied in that people in different regions of East, West, North and South have different customs, living habits, and characteristics of personality, and that seasons of spring, summer, autumn and winter influence body constitutions and the tendency for disease. People with more yang tend to be manic, while people with more yin tend to be depressed. Those are recorded in detail in *The Inner Canon of the Yellow Emperor* (*Huáng Dì Nèi Jīng*, 黄帝内经).

(5) REPRESENTATIVE FIGURES OF FIVE-STATUS CLASSIFICATION

1) People of Greater Yin: LIN Daiyu. She is sensitive and sentimental, who thinks deeply and carefully. This kind of people are prone to mental and physical health issues, and they are susceptible to mental illness and psychosomatic disorders.

2) People of Lesser Yin: SHA Monk. On the journey to the West for Buddhist scriptures, he carried luggage and followed Master TANG Sanzang. He went wherever the master asked him to go, without any complaint. This kind of people are self-disciplined, conscientious, persistent, serious, and observant.

3) People of Lesser Yang: ZHU Bajie. ZHU Bajie is also a novel character. He is active, rash, capricious, witty, flexible and disorderly on the journey to the West, who prefers to move than to stay still. He has many facial expressions, who is curious about new things. But he does not think much, which is the opposite of LIN Daiyu with profound thoughts.

4) People of Greater Yang: LI Kui. He can stick to his own point of view, and dare to contradict others. He is independent, arrogant, competitive, aggressive, and agile, with his own mindset and behavior style.

5) People of Balanced Yin-Yang: ZHUGE Liang. He is calm, emotionally stable, and sophisticated, carrying gentleness.

Everyone has the five characteristics of Greater Yin, Lesser Yin, Greater Yang, Lesser Yang and Balanced Yin-Yang to some extent, but is featured by one of them.

Self-designed questionnaires and standardized rating scales can assist with clinical assessments. Both "Five-Status Personality Test" and "Five-Five Body Constitution Test" involve questionnaires. Typical questions can be asked to assess the exact situations of patients and visitors, which is a commonly used method for psychological diagnosis.

6.9 Design of Five-Status Personality Test

Five-Status Personality Test (formulated in 1988 and revised in 2008) was compiled by Xue Chongcheng and authors from China Academy of Chinese Medical Sciences. Based on TCM theory of yin-yang, "five-status classification" recorded in *The Inner Canon of the Yellow Emperor* (*Huáng Dì Nèi Jing*, 黄帝内经), and modern methods of psychological scale construction, the test was formulated according to international standards, as the first indigenous measure of personality assessment in China. It achieved test norms involving the overall situation in China, gender, age, educational background and occupation as well as situations in different regions. The test is widely accepted by scholars at home and abroad, and frequently used in clinical practice, scientific research and other fields.

The test consists of 6 subscales with 103 items in total, including a credibility scale of 8 items, a subscale of 20 items for Greater Yang, a subscale of 22 items for Lesser Yang, a subscale of 21 items for Lesser Yin, and a subscale of 10 items for Balanced Yin-Yang. 1 point is scored for "yes" of each question, and 0 point for "no." At last, the total score of each subscale will be counted. If the credibility scale is scored less than 5, it will be regarded as an invalid test because of the lack of credibility.

6.10 Definition of yin and yang in traditional Chinese medicine

Traditional Chinese medicine believes that yin and yang are a pair of attributes that restrict each other. Where there is yin, there is yang, and where there is yang, there is yin. It is in the best state when they are balanced. Patients with depression are people of Greater Yin, whose behavior styles are characterized by Yin.

The Divine Pivot (Líng Shū, 灵枢) · The Ties between Yin and Yang Qi and Sun and Moon reads "Yin and Yang are invisible." Therefore, yin and yang are abstract opposing properties. Yang represents the positive, initiative, enterprising, and bright aspects of things, while yin implies the opposite. Yin and yang can correspond to inhibition and excitation in the nervous system. From the above, personalities can be determined based on the proportion of yin to yang. Likewise, personalities can be determined based on the proportion of excitation to inhibition. Normally, there is no pure yin or pure yang. Likewise, under normal circumstances, excitation or inhibition does not exist alone in the nervous system. Therefore, five-status classification can be supported by modern physiology.

Yin and yang are interdependent and opposing, which are not concrete. In emotional experience, descriptions of being quick and strong pertain to Yang, while those of being slow and weak pertain to Yin. Yin and yang are of a general principle covering all things. Each personality can be generalized according to yin and yang, involving fast or slow, external or internal, strong or weak, obvious or implicit, sensitive or insensitive.

6.11 Classification of body constitutions

The body constitution is a special state which is relatively stable in function, structure and metabolism, formed on the basis of congenital conditions and influenced by environments during the process of growth, development and aging. It often determines specificity of physiological response, as well as susceptibility to pathogenic factors and disease. Body constitutions involve both physical and mental health, which only refer to physical health conditions in certain context. Therefore, the determinants of body constitutions involve various physiological characteristics that influence mental states, including age, gender, physique, organ structure, personality traits, physiological functions, metabolism, and immunity. Those factors have different significance based on the social environment where an individual has been living. The theory of body constitutions attaches importance to innate factors, especially the stable factors of heredity affecting individuals, as well as weight and morphology influencing mental states and behaviors.

TCM considers that a healthy person has balanced body constitution, which is described as "people with balance of yin and yang and intact body-mind" in *The Inner Canon of the Yellow Emperor (Huáng Dì Nèi Jīng, 黄帝内经)*. We sampled among healthy people and did a survey of tens of thousands of samples all over China. The results showed that most of them had balanced body constitution. The body constitutions of sampled people can be divided into 13 types including 4 types classified according to the deficiency and excess of yin and yang, 4 types classified according to the deficiency and excess of qi and blood, 4 types of phlegm, dampness, wind and dryness, classified based on TCM treatment experience, as well as the balanced body constitution.

Body constitution measurement is based on the norms of psychological measurement. Each body constitution is simplified so that it is easier to be identified. Based on specific situations, different body constitutions can combine as complex body constitutions of individuals. For example, Qi and blood are important to women, who are prone to deficiency of qi and blood, and Qi deficiency can lead to blood stasis. Therefore, qi deficiency, blood deficiency and blood stasis usually combine as a complex body constitution. Balanced body constitution can also involve the combination though. Some people have yin deficiency and yang heat, who score high in both yin deficiency and yang heat.

6.12 Design of Five-Five Body Constitution Test

Five-Five Body Constitution Test (formulated in 2008) is TCM measurement of body constitution, funded by Ministry of Science and Technology in China and developed by Professor XUE Chongcheng and I according to TCM theory and experience of experts. Based on TCM theories of Qi, blood, yin and yang, as well as its explanations of body functions and biological substances, the test divides body constitutions into 13 categories (including balanced body constitution, body constitution of yang-heat, body constitution of yin-cold, body constitution of yang deficiency, body constitution of yin deficiency, body constitution of dampness, body constitution of phlegm, body constitution of wind, body constitution of dryness, body constitution of Qi deficiency, body constitution of blood deficiency, body constitution of qi stagnation, and body constitution of blood stasis). The test has a total of 28 major questions, including 195 items. 1 point is scored for "yes" of each item, and 0 point for "no." With verification, the test is reliable, of content validity, construct validity and discriminant validity, as well as consistency and stability. Scores are counted based on different types of body constitution. Test results can involve combinations of body constitution, such as body constitution of yin deficiency with yang heat, body constitution of Qi and blood deficiency, body constitution of qi stagnation and blood stasis, body constitution of phlegm and dampness, body constitution of phlegm and heat, which are in accordance with the theories and clinical practice of traditional Chinese medicine.

6.13 Factors affecting body constitutions

(1) Genetic factors. Heredity cannot be changed, but eugenics and prenatal care are advocated. Couples can start health cultivation before preparing for pregnancy. Although genetic endowments cannot be chosen, people should get to know and actively avoid genetic defects.

(2) Age. With the growth of age, the metabolic efficiency and organ functions of human body would change, which are normal physiological phenomena.

(3) Emotional factors.

(4) Environmental factors.

(5) Health status.

(6) Gender, eating habits, work and leisure, etc.

We cannot control many factors that affect health, such as ageing, genetic endowment, and gender, but we can live a good lifestyle to improve health.

6.14 Body-mind Regulation System of Five-Status

Body-mind Regulation System of Five-Status is established based on Five-Status Personality Test and Five-Five Body Constitution Test, involving not only tests but also health regulation plans based on test results. Health regulation plans include:

1) psychotherapy for self-cultivation;

2) diet therapy for improving both mental and physical health;

3) exercises such as Qigong, sports, and dance, for overall health regulation;

4) music therapy such as listening and singing, for improving both mental and physical health. Besides, there are other methods for overall health regulation, including TCM medication, moxibustion, and physical therapy.

(1) Body-mind Regulation System of Five-Status (as shown in Figure 6-2) is an intelligent system for providing measurement, evaluation and health regulation plans, which obtained the software copyright in 2014. The system provides advice on psychotherapy, diet therapy, exercises, music therapy and other methods including TCM medication, acupuncture and moxibustion, manipulation and physical therapy, for self-cultivation and overall health regulation.

1) Psychotherapy. Let me take people of Greater Yang with body constitution of yin deficiency and yang hyperactivity as an example. The body constitution of

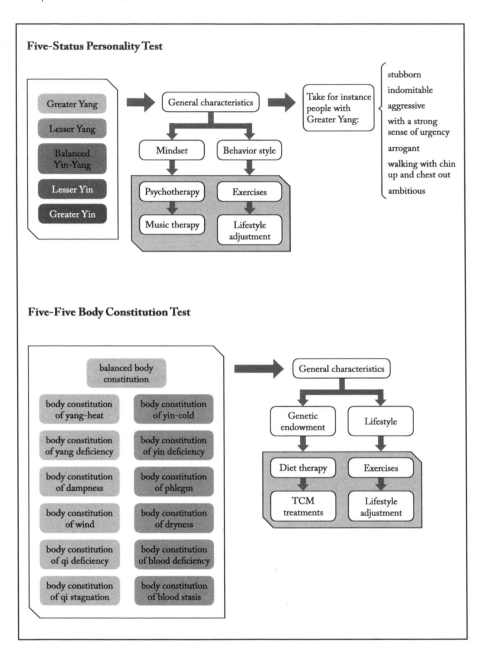

Figure 6-2   Body-mind Regulation System of Five-Status

yin deficiency and yang hyperactivity is positively correlated with the personality characteristics of Greater Yang, which embodies the concept of "intact body-mind" in traditional Chinese medicine. Physiologically, people of Greater Yang have more yang than yin. When yin is extremely low, the body constitution would be out of balance, so people of Greater Yang are unstable, active, irritable, emotional, stubborn, competitive, aggressive, and with a strong sense of urgency. The body constitution of yin deficiency and yang hyperactivity implies insufficient yin fluid and excessive yang heat, characterized by aversion to heat and preference for cold, liking for cold food, dry mouth, inflammation, dry stools, and thirst that cannot be quenched with drinking water. Such people can improve health with diet therapy, exercises and medication, because they have high metabolism. Psychotherapy can also help them raise awareness of psychology and ideology. It is difficult for them to persist in something beneficial for a long time due to lack of persistence. Therefore, people of Greater Yang should consciously control themselves and their emotions, who can do things as planned, avoid fuss over trifles, frequent arguments, or stubbornness, and listen to opinions of others to improve personality and stay calm. They are not recommended to attend competitive activities. Some people relax themselves through games. But people of Greater Yang are highly competitive when playing games, so games are energy-consuming to them, and their pursuit of high scores in games actually bring them the mental burden.

2) Diet therapy. Traditional Chinese medicine also puts emphasis on diet therapy. For example, Renshen (人参, Radix Ginseng), Goji berries, Hongdou Yimi Tang (红豆薏米汤, Red Beans and Semen Coicis Decoction) are great diet therapies for health preservation. Some people feel energetic after taking ginseng, but some people would have nosebleed and get irritable because they have different body constitutions. Different foods (or medicines) have different properties of being cold, heat, warm and cool, with different natures and tastes. Not all foods (or medicines) are suitable for everyone. For example, watermelons, bananas, and pears are fruits with cool property, which are suitable for people with the body constitution of heat, but not for those with the body constitution of cold. People with cold body constitution can have fruits with heat property, such as lychees, longans, and peaches. We must understand our body constitutions and get to know what foods are suitable for us, so that we can improve health with right diet therapies of appropriate amounts in proper ways. The foods that are not suitable for corresponding body constitutions should be avoided, which can be counterbalanced by foods of opposing properties if they are taken by chance, so as to keep balance and restore health.

3) Exercises. Different people like different sports. People of Greater Yang with body constitution of yin deficiency and yang hyperactivity would have Qi yin hurt after running with excessive sweating, which can aggravate yin deficiency and yang hyperactivity. Therefore, they are not suitable for strenuous exercise with fast rhythms, to whom gentle activities are recommended, such as Taijiquan, yoga and dance, to calm themselves down. Chinese square dancing is a good exercise, but it can lead to insomnia if people get too excited after dancing. Proper sports and music must be chosen to improve personality. When people of Greater Yang listen to the music with strong rhythm, they will be in high spirits, for whom relaxed music and folk music can help improve personality and calm them down. Besides, calligraphy is also beneficial. I knew a professor in Taiwan, whose nervous system was stimulated when he practiced calligraphy. His body and mind were coordinated during practice, which not only stimulated the brain through senses, but also regulated physical and mental health. Therefore, I think to practice calligraphy can not only benefit physical and mental health among healthy people, but also facilitate the recovery of hemiplegia patients and the elderly with cognitive dysfunction.

4) Environments. Some people have aversion to heat with liking for cool, so living conditions in summer must be adjusted to ensure comfort. People with the body constitution of yang heat live well in autumn and winter but have difficult time in spring and summer because weathers are cool in autumn and winter. People with the body constitution of yang deficiency and yin cold live well in spring and summer but have difficult time in autumn and winter, so they must take good care of themselves in autumn and winter. It can be seen that environmental factors must be paid attention to so as to avoid negative impacts of environments on human body.

5) Medical treatments. Appropriate medical treatments can improve physical and mental health. It should be noted that some people are not suitable for traditional moxibustion or electric moxibustion. Although moxibustion is a good method of health preservation, people with the body constitution of yin deficiency and yang heat are prone to inflammation after receiving moxibustion. If moxibustion is necessary during treatment, doctors should ask patients to drink more water and eat foods that can clear heat after receiving moxibustion. Otherwise, moxibustion may cause inflammation and sore throat, which would bring harm to body.

(2) SAMPLE CASE OF BODY-MIND REGULATION SYSTEM OF FIVE-STATUS.

Let's take people of Greater Yang with body constitution of yin deficiency and yang hyperactivity as an example.

1) Psychotherapy. Most people of Greater Yang have excessive yang, who are active and irritable. Therefore, they should increase self-cultivation and persistence training, improve personality to control feelings of excitement and irritability, learn to listen to others' opinions to avoid stubbornness or fuss over trifles, and avoid competitive activities.

2) Diet therapy. People of Greater Yang with body constitution of yin deficiency and yang hyperactivity should preserve yin to counter yang and stick to light and moistening diets. They can frequently eat sesame seeds, glutinous rice, honey, dairy products, fish, fruits and vegetables including balsam pears, tomatoes, cucumbers, lotus roots, grapes, bananas, watermelons, pears, pomelos, sugarcanes, persimmons, apples, but avoid spicy and dry foods, such as peppers, gingers, green onions, and have less foods that warm yang, such as beef, mutton, dog meat, chicken, and venison.

3) Exercises. Such people can practice Qigong and do sports, such as Taijiquan, Qigong of life cultivation, Qigong of health preservation, walking, jogging, playing balls, swimming, martial arts, Baduanjin, yoga, as well as gentle dance. It is not suitable for them to do exercises during the Chinese dog days of summer, because sweating in summer would aggravate yin deficiency and yang hyperactivity and hurt Qi yin, which would do harm to their body constitution.

4) Music. They can listen to peaceful and relaxing music, such as serenades and lullabies.

5) Environments. They have aversion to heat with liking for cool, who can live well in winter with cold weather but have difficult time in summer with hot weather, so they should be protected from heat in summer to take care of themselves.

6) Simple TCM medication. Chinese patent medicines can be taken according to doctor's advice and medication instructions. The dosage can be reduced if it is for health preservation in daily life.

7) Medicated diet. Medicines that are identified by national administration as foods can be taken to regulate health according to body constitutions, such as tremella fuciformis, bird nests, Dongchongxiacao (冬虫夏草, Cordyceps), Mohanlian (墨旱莲, Herba Ecliptae), Nu zhenzi (女贞子, Fructus Ligustri Lucidi), Shashen (沙参, Radix Adenophorae), Maidong (麦冬, Radix Ophiopogonis), Yuzhu (玉竹, Rhizoma Polygonati Odorati), and Baihe (百合, Bulbus Lilii).

8) Contraindications. Traditional moxibustion and electric moxibustion are not suitable for people with body constitution of yin deficiency and yang hyperactivity. If moxibustion is needed to relieve pain caused by wind-cold, patients can drink more water and eat foods that can nourish yin and clear heat after receiving moxibustion to avoid the harm moxibustion may bring to body.

Conclusion: it is significant to identify personalities and body constitutions no matter it is for clinical treatment or health preservation. Only after the characteristics of body and mind are identified can overall health regulation be made accordingly. Both physical health and mental health must be taken into consideration during clinical treatment and health preservation, then twice as much can be accomplished with half the effort. In TCM clinical treatment for psychosomatic disorders, syndrome differentiation and comprehensive treatment are adopted.

TCM medication (patent medicines or decoction) combined with acupuncture and moxibustion can be prescribed and psychological consulting can be recommended if necessary. Besides, patients need to live a healthy lifestyle. Then twice beneficial treatment results can be accomplished with half the effort. Therefore, my principle of treatment is to improve mental health for life cultivation and regulate mind for mental health preservation.

Five-Status Personality Test and Five-Five Body Constitution Test are the first standardized measure of mental and physical health assessment in TCM, which is a representative achievement in TCM psychology, making academic and practical contributions to the fields including clinical medicine, scientific research, medical education, healthcare management, and human resources.

Strengthening the Healthy Qi and Expelling the Evil Qi

Emotion Focused Therapies of Homeopathy in TCM

LECTURER: ZHANG BOHUA

Introduction to the speaker:

Zhang Bohua, PhD., is a professor, licensed TCM physician, and registered psychologist. She is a famous TCM psychologist who created the emotion focused therapies of homeopathy in traditional Chinese medicine. She is the founder of psychology discipline in Shandong University of traditional Chinese medicine, and the leader of TCM psychology of National Administration of Traditional Chinese Medicine in China. She is a TCM doctor and psychologist in Zhonglu Hospital affiliated to Shandong University of traditional Chinese medicine, and the chief in Baihualin Psychological Studio. Besides, Prof. Zhang is also the vice president of the specialty committee of TCM psychology of the World Federation of Chinese medicine Societies.

When I discussed with my friends about TCM psychology, they had many questions. What contributions does traditional Chinese medicine make to TCM psychology? What is the thought in TCM psychology? What are the therapies of TCM psychology and how can they be practiced? Can we still practice them today? Actually, many people have those questions, especially when Western models of psychotherapy are taken as the mainstream nowadays. A saying by Wang Yangming occurred to me, when I was thinking about the answer to those questions. "You give up endless treasures but take a bowl to beg from others."

Today, when people have psychological disorders, they may rely on external force to solve problems and seek treatment from others. But Wang Yangming believed that internal regulation of the mind was the most important, rather than external force of treatment. All the reason, wisdom, healthy emotions and the way to deal with them lied in your "mind." There were endless treasures hidden in your mind, but you didn't realize it and begged treatment from others. It may not be appropriate to use the idea of Wang Yangming to sum up the current situation of counseling psychology. But, isn't there a lack of something in counseling psychology today? Western models of psychotherapy spread widely and successfully in China, which benefits the mental health of people a lot indeed. However, traditional Chinese culture with a history of thousands of years is a great treasure. It seems we do not have much passion for it, but there are many precious ideas we can explore.

I put forward TCM emotion focused therapies of homeopathy in 2006. But it does not have an exact definition so far. Emotion focused therapies of homeopathy constitute a system with theories and skills, which is based on TCM theories, involving strengthening the healthy qi and expelling the evil qi, homeopathic remedies, yin-yang and five elements, as well as visceral emotions.

Besides TCM theories, emotion focused therapies of traditional Chinese medicine also apply TCM technology to treatment, such as the therapy of counteracting emotions. Some modern Western psychotherapies are also integrated into the therapy of counteracting emotions, including skills of communication and noncommunication. In clinical practice, therapies should be chosen according to the change and development of psychological states in patients (or visitors). Along with the course of treatment, emotions develop in different stages. Emotions that do harm to mental and physical health are regarded as stagnated emotions. To go with the flow of stagnated emotions is to tackle a complicated problem in an easy manner. Its effects can be summed up by a Chinese word "合和 (integrity and harmony)." "合" means integrity. In "和," the left part of "禾" means grains and the right part of "口" means mouth, which implies that harmony is reached when there is no lack of food and everyone is satisfied. Specifically, emotion focused therapies of homeopathy are to balance emotions, to regulate mental and physical health, and to maintain harmony between humans and nature. In short, there are a few important aspects of the therapies, including their theories, application, effects and targets.

7.1 Theories of emotions in TCM and their application

7.1.1 Understanding of emotions

Emotions are "情志" in Chinese. However, in ancient Chinese medical literature, there was no "情 (feeling)" at the beginning, but only "志 (ambition)." It is described that ambitions include "joy, anger, pensiveness, anxiety, and fear" in *Basic Questions (Sù Wèn, 素问) · Comprehensive Discourse on Arrangements of the Principal Qi of Heaven* and *Basic Questions (Sù Wèn, 素问) · Comprehensive Discourse on the Progression of the Five Periods*, in which pensiveness is in the middle. However, it is mentioned that five ambitions include "joy, anger, sorrow, anxiety, and fear" in *Basic Questions (Sù Wèn, 素问) · Comprehensive Discourse on Phenomena Corresponding to Yin and Yang.* There are also other statements about the five ambitions.

According to *Treatise on Diseases, Patterns, and Formulas Related to the Unification of the Three Etiologies (Sān Yīn Jí Yī Bìng Zhèng Fāng Lùn, 三因极一病证方论)* by Chen Wuze in Song dynasty, the factors affecting health can be divided into three categories in TCM, namely internal factors, external factors, and factors neither internal nor external. Seven feelings belong to internal factors, including joy, anger, anxiety, pensiveness, sorrow, fear, and shock. The seven feelings evolved from *The Inner Canon of the Yellow Emperor (Huáng Dì Nèi Jīng, 黄帝内经)*, but it can also be reduced to "five ambitions." Anxiety and sorrow are in the same category, which can be reduced to sorrow in the five ambitions; fear and shock are in the same category, which can be reduced to fear. Therefore, the "seven feelings" in the saying by Zhang Jingyue that "there are seven feelings in the world" actually correspond to the five ambitions in *The Inner Canon of the Yellow Emperor (Huáng Dì Nèi Jīng, 黄帝内经)*.

Zhang Jingyue put forward the concept of "emotional disease" in Ming dynasty. He summarized the discussions of emotion in *The Inner Canon of the Yellow Emperor (Huáng Dì Nèi Jīng, 黄帝内经)*. There is a treatise on stagnation syndrome in *The Complete Works of Zhang Jing-yue (Jǐng Yuè Quán Shū, 景岳全书)*, which sums up the three most common stagnation, namely anger stagnation, pensiveness stagnation and anxiety stagnation. Anger happens when something that you want to do cannot be done, and you are obstructed; pensiveness is about thinking without understanding and you cannot let it go. Anger and anxiety can be reduced to "thinking." Anxiety is about being unhappy, implying depression. So, what can be the treatment for the three types of stagnation? He said that "emotional disorders have to be dealt with emotions." A lot of people have emotional disorders today. What can help? Emotions themselves. It points to the importance of psychotherapy. According to Zhang Jingyue, if patients are woman, their wishes must be satisfied, and then emotions can be released. Anger dominating pensiveness can also help, but it only works temporarily and does not really solve the problem. Therefore, for females, only after their wishes are satisfied can their emotional stagnation be relieved. What if the patient is male? Zhang Jingyue said, "wise people with broadened minds are not easily attacked by the evil." As the old saying goes, "women are in charge of internal affairs in a family, while men work and make money to support the family." Therefore, men need to explore the world and do business. They must have a broad horizon. To what extent? In *Basic Questions* (*Sù Wèn*, 素问) · *Discourse on the True Qi Endowed by Heaven in High Antiquity*, it is said that people are interlinked with the spirit of heaven and earth. People who are truly inclusive do not worry any more. Therefore, for the diagnosis and treatment of the three stagnation syndromes, Zhang Jingyue put forward such a principle of gender differentiation, and put emphasis on psychology. In addition, traditional Chinese medicine stresses the unity of body and mind. Besides psychological treatment, Zhang Jingyue also prescribe medications to treat emotional disorders. For example, anger harms the liver, for which the formulas, including Jiegan San (解肝散, Powder for Relieving The Liver), Shenxiang San (神香散, Powder of Aromas), Liuyu Tang (六郁汤, Decoction for Six Stagnations) and Yueju Wan (越鞠丸, Depression-Resolving Pill), can help. If there is liver fire, formulas to nourish yin and clear heat such as Huagan Jian (化肝煎, Liver-Soothing Decoction) can be used. If anger lasts for a long time, it can cause phlegm, for which Wendan Tang (温胆汤, Gallbladder-Warming Decoction) can be prescribed.

In conclusion, *The Inner Canon of the Yellow Emperor* (*Huáng Dì Nèi Jing*, 黄帝 内经) discusses "ambitions." In Ming and Qing dynasties, the concept of emotions was highlighted and clinical practice involving psychotherapy was emphasized. Traditional Chinese medicine names the psychotherapy as emotion focused therapies. Emotions do not equate to feelings. In general psychology, feelings and sentiments are attitudes towards objective reality. Feelings are more related to whether people's biological needs are met, while sentiments, such as morality, are related to whether people's social needs are met. However, the emotions in TCM involve both feelings and ambitions. So, emotions are different from feelings. And emotions include emotional cognition.

7.1.2 The characteristics of emotions

(1) EMOTIONS HAVE THEIR OWN FEATURES.

Traditional Chinese medicine is a part of the extensive and profound Chinese traditional culture. In the history of ancient Chinese thought and philosophy, there is little discussion on emotions. The various schools of thought and their exponents discuss more about desires during the period from pre-Qin times to the early years of Han dynasty. For example, the saying by Guan Zhong that "when there is no lack of things, people know etiquette; when there are enough food and clothing, people know honor and disgrace" is more about desires. In the history of Chinese psychology, there is a special content about "the theory of desire," which records the thought about desires in the past dynasties, but there is little elaboration of emotions. Therefore, the concept of emotions and related theories are mainly discussed in traditional Chinese medicine. Of course, traditional Chinese medicine also talks about desires. For example, *Basic Questions (Sù Wèn, 素问) · Discourse on the True Qi Endowed by Heaven in High Antiquity* reads "when the sages of high antiquity taught those below, they always spoke to them about the following, that for the depletion evil and the robber wind, there are specific times when to avoid them; if there are quiet peacefulness and absolute emptiness, the true qi would follow." Quiet peacefulness and absolute emptiness are restraint of desires. There were four medical schools in Jin and Yuan dynasties. Zhu Danxi promoted nourishing yin. He thought that "yang is often surplus, while yin is often insufficient." "Surplus yang" implies desires with the restless mind. Yang pertains to motion, and moving leads to the consumption of minds as well as qi and blood. Sexual desire will inevitably consume energy, such as nocturnal emission and ejaculation. Therefore, "surplus yang" will harm yin, leading to "insufficient yin is often."

(2) EMOTIONS HAVE THE CHARACTERISTIC OF HOLISM.

Firstly, emotions and zang-fu organs interrelate. The five qi of zang organs generate emotions. According to *Basic Questions (Sù Wèn, 素问) · Comprehensive Discourse on Arrangements of the Principal Qi of Heaven*, people have five zang organs, namely heart, liver, spleen, lung and kidney. The physiological function of five zang organs is called qi transformation. Emotions result from the qi transformation in organs. Traditional Chinese medicine holds that emotions are the external manifestation of qi transformation in five zang organs, including joy, anger, pensiveness, anxiety, and fear. Some people may ask, can we apply this idea to psychotherapy and psychosomatic health services today? It is worth thinking about. In my view, it is important to explore how emotions come into being. As Wang Yangming said, seeking from the inside is to explore the reasons for the formation of emotions. But does the inside refer to biology or psychology? It is also a question. Actually, we can seek not only from the inside, but also from the outside.

The generation of emotions and the influence of emotions on zang-fu organs show that emotions and zang-fu organs are closely related. Emotions can be used for treatment. A case of Zhu Danxi was recorded in *Complete Records of Medical Works* (*Yī Bù Quán Lù*, 医部全录) by Chen Menglei in Qing dynasty. A female had little news about her newly married husband who had been in Guang City for five years, so facing the north, she was bedridden with no appetite. It is regarded that anxiety and pensiveness harm the spleen. Please think about how emotions affect zang-fu organs in treatment. Zhu Danxi used the method of anger dominating pensiveness to treat. Then she had appetite and could eat.

I also had a clinical case.

There was a 60-year-old man from the countryside. When I asked him what was wrong, he grabbed his throat and said that he had not eaten for a month. Isn't it contradictory? How could he stay alive and come to see a doctor if he had not eaten for a month? I asked him again what he had if he hadn't eaten for a month. He said he drank juice, but he couldn't swallow it. There was something in his throat, with difficulty swallowing. I asked whether he went to the department of gastroenterology. He said that all the examinations had been done, and everything was ok, so the doctor in the department of gastroenterology asked him to see a psychologist. He kept trying to swallow. Observed from the lateral, when he was swallowing, the larynx moved up and down difficultly, especially when it moved downward. He said he had difficulty swallowing. But what difficultly, especially when it moved downward. He said he had difficulty swallowing. But what did he swallow? I said, "bro, you have a grievance." He didn't get it and asked me again. And I repeated, "you have a grievance." His tears came down immediately after hearing that. My words hit the crux of the matter. Then, he cried and began to tell his story. When he finished the story, he aired his grievance. It was about the emotion focused therapy of homeopathy. To go with the flow of stagnated emotions is to tackle a complicated problem in an easy manner. He spoke everything out and finally saw the hope of life. And I prescribed no medication during that treatment. Two weeks later, his son came to me and said that his father had eaten noodles after the treatment, and his appetite was improved. So, this case shows that the relationship between emotions and zang-fu organs is inseparable. The so-called TCM emotion focused therapies are based on the theories of traditional Chinese medicine, to firstly understand physical symptoms, and then release emotions, so as to restore health.

Secondly, emotions and thinking (cognition) are interrelated. *The Inner Canon of the Yellow Emperor* (*Huáng Dì Nèi Jīng*, 黄帝内经) has a very good description of the cognitive process of human beings, "those who know the heaven well must understand people; those who know history well must understand the present; those who know Qi well must understand things." That is to say, cognition must be tested by practice. Cognition starts from perception. Then, thinking is to understand the internal laws of things, and after that, it goes into consideration. In ancient epistemology, consideration is a deeper cognitive activity than thinking. After consideration, it rises to rational cognition, and then returns to practice for verification. It is about cognition. The relationship between emotions and thinking can be important for diagnosis and for the practice of TCM emotion focused therapies of homeopathy.

Thirdly, emotions and nature are interrelated. By far, Western psychotherapy puts little emphasis on the relationship between human psychology and nature, and few doctors use this relationship to improve mental health. Horticultural therapy only involves planting flowers and grasses, which is far less abundant than the contents in traditional Chinese medicine.

What is the relationship between "unity of nature and human" and emotion focused therapies of homeopathy? It stresses going with the flow of stagnated emotions. But how do emotions happen and develop? Related factors include cognition, zang-fu organs and the environment. Therefore, that is to go with the flow of factors that affect emotions, which is the embodiment of "unity of nature and human."

What is the relationship between nature and our mind and body? *The Divine Pivot* (*Líng Shū*, 灵枢) reads, "heaven manifests itself within me as virtue; the earth manifests itself within me as qi; when the virtue flows and the qi have joined, life begins," so human life (being alive) and all things are born between heaven and earth. What is life? Life is being alive and where we live is between heaven and earth. What is qi? Qi implies change. In early spring, green leaves grow, which implies "the earth within me." "Those who know Qi well must understand things." That is to say, the change of qi is manifested by the change of things. "Heaven manifests itself within me as virtue; the earth manifests itself within me as qi." There are the sun, rain and dew, wind, frost, rain and snow in the heaven. They generate everything and people between heaven and earth. Therefore, "with the qi of heaven, tranquility will govern the mind." The governance does not mean the activity of governing, but it implies the overall normality of the world. "Sages with the qi of heaven understand everything and pass on the spirit." That is to say, sages know the relationship between human and nature very well, so they can inherit the spirit of heaven and earth, and then practice according to the law of nature.

Therefore, we should obtain the positive energy from nature to cultivate and strengthen the mind, and deal with dissatisfaction in dialectical ways. Nature not only supports us to live, but also restrain us.

"Great virtue carrying things" implies nature nurtures all things. People like to see the fields full of hope. When you look at this scene, do you just look at the green or just enjoy the scenery? It is also about understanding the humanistic spirit of "great virtue carrying things," which implies "unity of nature and human." Therefore, the integrity of emotions includes the integrity of emotions and zang-fu organs, the integrity of feelings and ambitions, as well as the close relationship between emotions and nature.

7.2   Emotion focused therapies

7.2.1   Psychological counseling in TCM

Is there psychological counseling in traditional Chinese medicine? How does it work? *Basic Questions (Sù Wèn, 素问) · Comprehensive Discourse on Phenomena Corresponding to Yin and Yang* reads, "those who know the heaven well must understand people; those who know history well must understand the present; those who know Qi well must understand things." That is to say, cognition must be tested by practice. Yin and yang are abstract, used to describe things. For the liver, "the ambition of liver is anger," which means anger harms the liver. But what can help with the "liver injury"? What can relieve anger? Sorrow dominates anger. Can joy dominate anger? Yes. So, when reading *Inner Canon of the Yellow Emperor (Huáng Dì Nèi Jīng, 黄帝内经)*, we must understand the contents comprehensively. For the heart, "the ambition of heart is joy." Joy harms the heart, but in what way? Joy dissipates the heart qi. For example, difficulty in concentrating implies the dissipation of heart qi, which means the heart is hurt. What can help with the "heart injury"? Fear dominates joy. For the spleen, "the ambition of spleen is pensiveness." If a person tends to split hairs, anger can help. For example, some patients with mental illness would have hallucinations if they concentrate the mind because they tend to split hairs. Therefore, in clinical practice, I try to broaden their minds and distract their attention from details. The lung corresponds to anxiety, so anxiety harms the lung. Joy dominates anxiety. For the kidney, "the ambition of kidney is fear." When frightened, patients can be incontinent in a state of utter stupefaction, which implies the kidney is hurt. Pensiveness dominates fear. This is about the therapy of counteracting emotions. In Jin and Yuan dynasties, the therapy of counteracting emotions developed well, which had great therapeutic effects and could be managed properly in different ways even if side effects occurred in clinic. Medications can hardly benefit the stagnation caused by emotions, so psychotherapies are necessary. The therapy of counteracting emotions is actually a very simple representative.

7.2.2 Personal understanding of emotions

Traditional ideas of emotions bring me inspiration. Take fear as an example. Fear is a feeling. But what exactly are we frightened of? The things we fear are transformed into the "impression" in our mind. We perceive words, sights, sounds, etc. Sights include characters and images, which are components of cognition. Besides, concepts are also present in the mind. For example, we often have fear, disgust and other feelings at caterpillars, which are components of sentiments. At the same time, the body may feel itchy. Different individuals can have different physical feelings though. Disgust and fear imply feelings of aversion and nausea. Nausea is a physical symptom. Fear brings about avoidance, which is also a physical component. When the three components come together, emotions happen as the integrity. The components of cognition, sentiment and the body contribute to the response to a stimulus. There is another example. A Chinese saying goes that "lotus flowers out of the mud refuse to be contaminated," which describes the noble personality. This is about Chinese culture, which is implicit with many connotations. Lotus flowers grow up in sludge, but they stay clean, elegant, and beautiful. So, in Chinese culture, the connotation of a lotus is noble personality. Then, emotions can come after understanding the culture. When you see a lotus, the impression in your mind would remind you if its concept, which contributes to the cognitive component. Feeling comfortable and refreshed mentally after seeing the lotus is a component of sentiment, and then the body will also feel refreshed and comfortable, which is the physical component. Therefore, in my view, emotions happen based on the three components.

7.2.3 Three components of emotions

Sentiments usually come with cognition. The three components are combined when emotions happen. In general, before I practice emotion focused therapies of homeopathy, I identify sentiments to determine whether they are simple or complex, mild or severe, conscious or unconscious, lasting long or short. Then I would study the specific event. Besides, the physical component can be a symptom. When visitors come to us, we observe them first. Some have strong feelings, through which we can analyze cognitive and physical components. It is very common. Some present with more physical symptoms. They may have dysphagia, poor appetite, headache, nausea, vomiting, constipation, chest tightness, abdominal pain, leg pain, weakness of limbs, etc. Usually, people with those symptoms will go to the hospital, but they cannot be cured, so doctors would advise them to see psychologists. Such cases are less frequently seen in a psychological outpatient clinic, or a psychological counseling center, compared with the general outpatient clinic. Those symptoms can be caused by feelings. For example, the patient with difficulty swallowing mentioned above had the feeling of grievance. But he might not have realized the connection between difficulty swallowing and grievance and might not have noticed his sentiment of grievance. What's more, the cognitive component implied by symptoms could be hidden even deeper. Anyway, the physical symptoms and sentiments that you can be aware of, as well as hidden cognitive components, are all integrated as emotions, but they can be present in different ways.

The three components of emotions are of great significance in psychological counseling. No matter how emotions are expressed, I always bear in mind that there are cognitive components and physical components (i.e., body sense) behind sentiments. This way of thinking is very helpful to make a diagnosis. If patients have more obvious physical components, I would also look for their components of cognition and sentiments, based on the integrity of emotions. Therefore, it is a process of psychological evaluation and diagnosis.

7.2.4 The thought of strengthening the healthy qi and expelling the evil qi

Traditional Chinese medicine believes that there are two basic forces in the process of disease development, that is, the healthy qi and the evil qi, corresponding to positive energy and negative energy. They compete with each other. Therefore, in the whole process of disease development, there are several states in the contest between the two forces, including abundant evil qi with deficient healthy qi; prevailing healthy qi with retreating evil qi; evil qi equal to healthy qi; deficient healthy qi with remnants of evil qi.

The four states are related to the recovery and aggravation of disease. The competition between healthy and evil forces is also important for psychotherapy. When the positive energy is strong, the negative energy will retreat and mental problems will be improved. If the negative energy prevails, mental illness will be aggravated. So, what is the evil qi in psychology? It refers to the events that disturb and upset the mind, leading to stagnated emotions. What is the healthy qi in psychology? It refers to the power that restores inner peace, which implies the self-healing, self-motivated and potential mental ability. In short, two forces of psychology are the evil qi of stagnated emotions, and the healthy qi of self-healing power.

Parents of many visitors also have mental problems. They are too anxious about the problems of their children. If you only look at problems (evil), the evil qi will be strengthened. If you look forward to the healthy qi, it will also be improved. At the beginning of treatment, the evil qi prevails, so stagnated emotions are manifested by intense symptoms. At this time, the priority is to eliminate pathogenic factors. After the evil qi is dispelled, the healthy qi is enhanced, with positive energy equal to negative energy, or with recovered healthy qi. Then, the treatment is to expel evil qi and reinforce healthy qi. In the late stage of treatment, the healthy qi is superior to the evil qi, so healthy qi can be further strengthened. This is about the principle of psychological counseling, during which we should take into account both the negative and the positive forces.

7.2.5 The thought of TCM emotion focused therapies of homeopathy

(1) THE FLOW OF EMOTIONS

Basic Questions (*Sù Wèn*, 素问) · *Comprehensive Discourse on Phenomena Corresponding to Yin and Yang* reads "when a disease begins to emerge, one can pierce and the disease ends." That is to say, at the beginning of disease, it is mild. What can we do? "Piercing" implies moderate treatment. "When it abounds, one must wait until it weakens and the disease, when pierced, ends." It means when the disease is severe, we should follow the flow of its forces, and give treatment after the disease declines. "Hence, after it has become light, scatter it. After it has become heavy, eliminate it. When it is on high, trace it and disperse it. When it is down below, pull and eliminate it." When a problem is located at the upper part of the body, treatments of guiding downward, such as diuresis and defecation, will not be used. For problems located at the upper part, such as coughing, volatile leafy or herbal medicine, such as Suye (苏叶, Folium Perillae) and Bohe (薄荷, Herba Menthae), can be used. If a problem is located in the lower part of the body, such as the problems of urination and defecation, medications of guiding downward can be used, such as Fuling (茯苓, Poria) and Dahuang (大黄, Radix et Rhizoma Rhei). This is about the idea of homeopathy, to go with the flow of disease. *The Divine Pivot* (*Líng Shū*, 灵枢) · *The Transmissions from the Teachers* reads "one should see to it that one acts in accordance with the expectations of all the people, the entire population," which also embodies the thought of homeopathy in psychology. In the early stage of emotion focused therapies of homeopathy, evil qi prevails, so to let it go is important. In the middle and late stages, the evil qi declines and then treatment can be given accordingly.

(2) THE OBJECT OF EMOTION FOCUSED THERAPIES

Every psychotherapy has its own treatment object. TCM emotion focused therapies of homeopathy target stagnated emotions. Stagnation implies a blockage and a mess in the mind. As the saying goes, "a heart has thousands of blockages." They can come into being in a short period of time or by years. Some blockages occur all of sudden, caused by intense stimuli.

(3) EMOTIONAL COGNITION

According to Zhang Jiebin, "seven emotions derive from likes and dislikes." Likes and dislikes are mental prerequisites, which indicates that the tendencies have existed for a long time. Sentiments like disgust, envy, doubt, and fear are underlying. Therefore, once something that you hate appear, underlying sentiments will be revealed. Therefore, such cognition is always there, underlying or subconscious, which can be seen not only in disease but also in dreams.

(4) PHYSICAL FEELING OF EMOTIONS

Take headache as an example. Headache is a pun. In one way, it really means headache, when patients are complaining that "my temples hurt," "my forehead hurts," and "my head aches." In the other way, when you encounter insurmountable difficulties, you will also have a headache. For another example, when the throat feels blocked, it is called foreign body sensation, with the difficulty of vomiting and swallowing.

Functional discomforts without organic disease are regarded as the disorders of qi mechanism in TCM. Qi goes up and down, and moves inward and outward. When your qi is in disorder, its movement will be messed up. Failure of vomiting and defecation can be the manifestation of the disorder. Sneezing and blowing the nose are also the external manifestation of internal qi disorder, which reflects the relationship between mind and body. Those are what we call physical feelings or symptoms, which can be described specifically by qi going up and down, qi alleviation, qi stagnation and qi disorder.

(5) ASSESSMENT OF STAGNATED EMOTIONS

The assessment of stagnated emotions goes through the whole process of emotion focused therapies, and it is very flexible. Emotions are changeable because humans are complicated. Joy can turn into sorrow, and anxiety can come with fear. Therefore, emotional assessment is necessary in psychological counselling. The cognitive components of stagnated emotions can be conflicts or events, which must be analyzed. Also, physical components of stagnated emotions have their own features, which also need to be identified. In the process of evaluation, it is also necessary to evaluate the mental resources and find out where the mental resources are from.

(6) EXPRESSION OF STAGNATED EMOTIONS

There are many ways to express stagnated emotions, such as language, imitation, and behaviors. Many of them are unique in traditional Chinese medicine. There are sound therapies of tones including jue, zhi, gong, shang, and yu, physical therapies such as manipulation and massage, body graffiti, etc. Imitation can also be used in psychotherapy. For example, there are movements of Taijiquan. Every set of movement has a name. When you practice the movement of seeking a needle at the bottom of the sea, you would imagine looking for a needle in the sea and you would start to concentrate. When you practice the movement of white crane spreading wings, you will feel extended and relaxed. Every movement has its connotation and requires imagination.

Physical symptoms and the mental state are linked. It can be embodied in treatment. Take body graffiti as an example. When you have chest tightness, you can draw a head with a circle and the chest with other shapes under the head. Then, you scrawl on them, and gradually stagnation will be relieved. Actually, during drawing and scrawling, inner stagnation is expressed out. For headache, leg pain, and low back pain, you can also do this. That process has another function, during which sudden enlightenment may occur and stagnated emotions are released.

Therapeutic Solutions

Introduction to Emotion Focused Therapies of Traditional Chinese Medicine

LECTURER: LI ZHAOJIAN

Introduction to the speaker:

Li Zhaojian, with a PhD in medicine, is a research fellow, licensed physician, psychotherapist, and counseling psychologist. He studied in Shanghai Mental Health Center for 2 years, and received training in *"Sino-German Psychoanalytic Psychotherapy Training Program"* and *"Sino-American Cognitive Behavior Therapy Training Program"* from 2005 to 2010. Prof. Li commits himself to the clinical practice of integrated Chinese and Western medicine, and actively advocates maintaining mental and physical health by means of traditional culture. He has been engaged in researches on psychosomatic medicine since 1995, and broke into psychological counseling in 1998.

Humans have various and complicated psychological phenomena. Psychological factors are responsible for the occurrence, development, and outcome of many diseases. Psychology somewhat links social factors to physiology and pathology, and thus psychological and social factors can be causes of disease. For psychogenic illnesses and psychosomatic diseases, medications are often found not working well or even ineffective, while non-medication treatments have positive effects. Therefore, illness such as psychological disorders, psychosomatic diseases, neuropsychiatric diseases, and maladaptive behaviors also require psychological treatments aimed at managing relapses and maintaining health, in addition to relieving symptoms by means of internal medicine.

Psychotherapy has existed at home and abroad since ancient times, but it did not have systematic theories and techniques then. In the past 40 years, its importance has increasingly been recognized by the medical community. People have conducted research on psychotherapy and made it into the fourth treasure of modern medicine to treat disease. Psychotherapy is a complex and important subject, covering a wide range of aspects. Therefore, there are more difficulties in studying and practicing psychotherapy, compared to other medical treatments.

Currently, psychotherapy does not have an accepted and clear definition. But academia believes that psychotherapy is a special interpersonal communication. In short, it involves a special interpersonal relationship. No matter whether a drug is used or not, from a broad perspective, psychotherapy include any methods that can affect emotions so as to improve treatment effects, also known as psychotherapy for mental illnesses.

At present, domestic psychotherapy is mostly based on Western theories of psychology, which is deeply influenced by Western culture and Western social customs. Although such psychotherapy is more rigorous in treatment planning, with advanced methods and strong evidence, it still has geographical restrictions. The psychological phenomena in people of different nationalities and different cultures have many similarities, but there are many differences in their types, properties, features and so on. The social culture in China is different from that of the West in historical evolution, cultural tradition, social structure, economic conditions, values, lifestyle and social customs, etc. Personality traits and psychological states of Chinese people are also very different from those of westerners. Chinese people have their special psychological problems and mental disorders. Cultural differences are also reflected in the situations that Chinese and Western people often have different specific causes and symptoms even for the same type of psychological problems and psychiatric disorders. Based on the above factors, Western theories and treatments cannot be rigidly applied to psychotherapy because there is no such an omnipotent system of psychotherapy in the world, not even in the future.

British scholar Jane Ogden believes that "personality, behavior, religious belief, and social environment are leading causes of disease." Confucianism, Buddhism, and Taoism are important spiritual wealth of the Chinese nation. For thousands of years, Chinese culture has deeply influenced Chinese people, physically and mentally. Confucianism, Taoism, and Buddhism are abundant in the theories and methods of maintaining "mind and body at ease" to restore health. Traditional Chinese medicine (TCM) is deeply rooted in traditional culture, absorbing nutrients from Confucianism, Buddhism, and Taoism. As a medical science, TCM made great contributions to maintaining physical and mental health for Chinese people. TCM is a good entry point to explore psychological barriers, psychosomatic diseases and so on in the inherent cultural background of China. Putting emphasis on mental health has been a feature and advantage of TCM characterized by holism and overall regulation. In the long-term development of TCM, it created many unique psychological therapies with rich experience, which basically agree with the definition, methods and effects of modern psychotherapy. TCM psychotherapy, based on traditional Chinese culture, is more suitable for the personality traits of Chinese people.

There is no such term as psychology or psychotherapy in TCM, but there are many similar expressions in ancient literatures. The well-known ones are "regulating the spirit" from *The Inner Canon of the Yellow Emperor: Basic Questions (Huáng Dì Nèi Jīng Sù Wèn,* 黄帝内经素问) · *Discourse on Treasuring Life and Preserving Physical Appearance*, "regulating the mind" from *Supplement to 'Classified Case Records of Famous Physicians' (Xù Míng Yī Lèi Àn,* 续名医类案), "treating the heart" from *Secret records of life cultivation (Qīng Náng Mì Lù,* 青囊秘录), "restraining oneself" from *Teachings of [Zhu] Dan-xi (Dān Xī Xīn Fǎ,* 丹溪心法), etc.

TCM psychotherapy generally refers to language, behavior, specially arranged scenes and so on, affecting emotions, instead of "tangible" treatments such as drugs, acupuncture, or surgery. Those can bring positive energy into patients to prevent disease and restore health, improving physical and mental performance. Some "mind therapies" and "heart therapies" are performed in conjunction with acupuncture and medications, which is similar to Western psychotherapy. A large number of clinical practices have proved that the therapeutic effects can complement each other if psychotherapy is practiced together with acupuncture and medications.

Traditional Chinese medicine gathers experience of the Chinese nation in its long-term struggle against diseases. It has a unique theoretical system formed under the influence of ancient Chinese philosophical thoughts. TCM, as a science, studies physiology and pathology, guiding doctors to make diagnoses and prevent diseases through syndrome differentiation and treatment. Holism is embodied in abundant TCM psychological thoughts, which emphasizes that spirit, cognition, and mentalities are supported by internal organs. Individuals have significant differences in psychological activities, influenced by natural and social environments. TCM has rich experience in treating mental diseases. "Mental illness has to be dealt with mental approaches" is a well-known saying in China. Psychotherapy is actually one of the oldest methods of medical treatment, which was once of mainstream medicine in ancient times.

American scholar Murphy once said, "psychology originates from China." It is ascertained that *Formulas for Fifty-two Diseases* (*Wŭ Shí Èr Bìng Fāng*, 五十二病方) from the Mawangdui Silk Texts is an ancient medical text before *The Inner Canon of the Yellow Emperor* (*Huáng Dì Nèi Jīng*, 黄帝内经) came into being, which contains 35 medical cases of "Zhuyou exorcism." *The Inner Canon of the Yellow Emperor* (*Huáng Dì Nèi Jīng*, 黄帝内经), which came into being more than 2,000 years ago, is not only a collection of TCM theories, but also the oldest book on medical psychology. *The Inner Canon of the Yellow Emperor* recognizes that psychological factors are closely related to pathogenesis, disease course, and prognosis, in which "regulating the spirit" is placed at the top of various therapies, and treatment methods such as "acupuncture and medication" must be applied with proper mental status of patients to take effect. *The Divine Pivot* (*Líng Shū*, 灵枢) · *The Transmissions from the Teachers* reads "The intrinsic nature of humans is such: there is no one who does not abhor death and enjoys life. Inform them of what will destroy them. Tell them what will be good for them. Guide them to what will ease their condition. Open their minds to everything that will bring suffering. Even if these are people who do not follow the WAY, why should they not listen?" The incisive discourse is still considered as a typical theory of psychology. *Basic Questions* (*Sù Wèn*, 素问) · *Comprehensive Discourse on the Progression of the Five Periods* and *Basic Questions* (*Sù Wèn*, 素问) · *Comprehensive Discourse on Phenomena Corresponding to Yin and Yang* recognize mental health and physical health can influence each other physiologically and pathologically and so can different emotions. Therefore, based on the principle of "counteracting," there came a unique treatment of "anger harms the liver; sadness dominates anger; joy harms the heart; fear dominates joy; pensiveness harms the spleen; anger dominates pensiveness; anxiety harms the lung; joy dominates anxiety; fear harms the kidneys; pensiveness dominates fear." *Basic Questions* (*Sù Wèn*, 素问) · *Discourse on Moving the Essence and Changing the Qi* records "When the people in antiquity treated a disease, they simply moved the essence and changed the qi. They were able to invoke the origin and any disease came to an end." That is, Zhuyou exorcism, invoking the origin, regulates the mental health condition, thereby changing the pathological state of qi and blood disorder. The so-called Zhuyou exorcism is a spiritual therapy through ritual performance to counter-balance emotions, which seeks to find out the cause of disease. In ancient times, there was the department of Zhuyou exorcism in hospital, which can be regarded as the beginning of TCM psychology. *Basic Questions* (*Sù Wèn*,

素问) · *Discourse on Strange Diseases* describes that "One severely scares the patient. That, too, may end the hiccup." and *Basic Questions (Sù Wèn, 素问) · Comprehensive Discourse on the Essentials of the Most Reliable* reads "what is scared, calm it," which reflect the practice of psychotherapy. *Basic Questions (Sù Wèn, 素问) · Discourse on the True [Qi Endowed by] Heaven in High Antiquity* reads "They exhaled and inhaled essence qi. They stood for themselves and guarded their spirit. Muscles and flesh were like one." *Basic Questions (Sù Wèn, 素问) · Discourse on Different [Therapeutic] Patterns Suitable [for Use in Different] Cardinal Points* records "guiding-pulling and pressing-lifting" and *Basic Questions (Sù Wèn, 素问) · Discussion on Acupuncture Methods* reads "tranquilizing the mind and eliminating avarice, holding the breath (only inhalation and no exhalation) for seven times," which advocates practicing Qigong to prevent disease, regulate the spirit, and restore health.

All in all, *Inner Canon of the Yellow Emperor (Huáng Dì Nèi Jīng, 黄帝内经)* has initially established the basic principles and techniques of TCM psychology, which still has a great influence on today. During the same period of that book, *Master Lvs Spring and Autumn Annals (Lǚ Shì Chūn Qiū, 吕氏春秋)* recorded that Doctor Wen Zhi treated King Qi Min with anger and was thus killed, and *The Chronicles of the Latter Han Dynasty (Hòu Hàn Shū, 后汉书)* recorded that Hua Tuo treated governors through irritating, which are well-known and complete medical cases of TCM psychotherapy.

Although *Treatise on Cold Damage (Shāng Hán Lùn, 伤寒论)* in the Han Dynasty did not explicitly propose a method of psychological treatment, Zhang Zhongjing clearly stated in *Essentials from the Golden Cabinet (Jīn Guì Yào Lüè, 金匮要略) · Pathogenesis of Disease Chapter One* that psychosomatic disorders should be taken into consideration during the treatment of disease.

During the Jin-Yuan period, there were a number of doctors who practiced psychotherapy well. *Confucians' Duties to Their Parents (Rú Mén Shì Qīn, 儒门事亲) · Diseases Caused by Nine Types of Qi* by Zhang Zihe is a monograph on psychotherapy, which interprets and develops the theories of emotion-focused therapy in *The Inner Canon of the Yellow Emperor (Huáng Dì Nèi Jīng, 黄帝内经)* and it makes a review about his innovative methods of psychotherapy. Psychological cases of Zhang Zihe are creditable in treatment planning, therapeutic approaches and the integrity of record. Those are high-level medical cases no matter from the perspective of traditional Chinese medicine or modern psychology, which are influential not only in China, but also in the historical development of psychotherapy worldwide. In the same age as Zhang zihe, Luo Tianyi, Zhu Danxi, Jia Sicheng, and other experts also documented cases of effective psychotherapy. It is worth noting that psychotherapy was not only used by Han nationality, but also by other ethnic groups in China. For example, Yelv Dilu in the Liao dynasty purged poison through infuriating in a treatment.

Miao Zhongchun in the Ming Dynasty thought "emotions derive from cognition, detectable but unpredictable; different situations can be emotional triggers, and it is hard to regulate if people are indulged in an emotion," and "emotional indulgence can happen repeatedly." For treatment, there is a discourse that "Cognitive restructuring and reasoning can be used to regulate emotions, because mental illness has to be dealt with mental approaches. Then, people getting rid of emotional triggers can overcome emotional disorders so as to remain self-possessed." In *The collection of Herbs* (*Běn Cǎo Jīng Shū*, 本草经疏) · *Volume 1 On Seven emotions*. Zhang Jingyue carried on the past and opened a way for future, interpreting and developing the theories of psychotherapy in *The Inner Canon of the Yellow Emperor* (*Huáng Dì Nèi Jīng*, 黄帝内经). He took the clinical psychology cases of his own and others as examples to profoundly analyze Zhuyou exorcism in *The Classified Classic* (*Lèi Jīng*, 类经) · *On Treatment*. Besides, *The Complete Works of [Zhang] Jing-yue* (*Jǐng Yuè Quán Shū*, 景岳全书) has made a historic contribution to the treatment of malingering. The fact is that most clinical cases of psychology were documented in the Ming Dynasty.

Rhymed Discourse on External Remedies (*Lǐ Yuè Pián Wén*, 理瀹骈文) by Wu Shangxian in the Qing Dynasty reads "medication cannot handle mental problems, so emotional disorders have to be treated with emotional approaches," which remains a well-known theory. There were only a few fragments of psychotherapy during that period, and psychotherapy was mostly taken as alternative treatment and performed in conjunction with acupuncture and medication. However, it still has a great significance on the collection of psychotherapy cases. There are more than 30 cases of psychological treatment in *Complete Records of Ancient and Modern Medical Works of the Grand Compendium of Books* (*Gǔ Jīn Tú Shū Jí Chéng Yī Bù Quán Lù*, 古今图书集成医部全录) by Chen Menglei and more than 20 cases in *Supplement to 'Classified Case Records of Famous Physicians'* (*Xù Míng Yī Lèi Àn*, 续名医类案) by Wei Zhixuan, which are monographs on psychotherapy, focusing on malingering, lovesickness and so on. Although *Comments on Ancient and Modern Case Records* (*Gǔ Jīn Yī Àn Àn*, 古今医案按) by Yu Zhen contains less psychotherapeutic cases, but it has higher quality and more incisive comments.

With abundant clinical experience, the past generations of doctors summed up that "mental illness has to be dealt with mental approaches," and put forward "mental illness could be treated with an unknown medication with mysterious properties, uncertain dosage and fascinating actions, produced in an undiscovered place." It can be seen that "mental approaches" are actually non-medication therapies, referring to psychotherapies. Zhao Yanxuan in the Qing dynasty clearly put forward in *Medical Notes of Cun Cun Zhai* (*Cún Cún Zhāi Yī Huà Gǎo*, 存存斋医话稿) that "emotionless herbs cannot cure emotion disorders, and intractable disease should be handled with eloquent speech." For doctors who do not attach importance to psychological treatment, there is a sharp criticism in *Precious Mirror of Oriental Medicine* (*Dōng Yī Bǎo Jiàn*, 东医宝鉴) that "The ancient sacred doctors, who can heal the mind, protected people from disease, while doctors nowadays can only treat disease but not take care of the mind, grasping the shadow instead of the essence. Isn't it foolish? Quack doctors only help with temporary relief, which is unpromising."

Overall therapeutic strategy is the basic content of holism in TCM, which has been limited to "tangible" treatment of acupuncture and medication for a long time, ignoring the "invisible" psychological treatment. Before the founding of the People's Republic of China, the study on TCM psychology could be found occasionally in TCM literatures, and most of the study focused on individual medical cases. Theoretical studies focused more on the cause and development of seven emotions, as well as pathogenesis, disease course, and prognosis of mental disorders. Since the 1980s, the study of TCM psychology has been active. Many scholars made significant explorations, which has not been widely paid attention to in TCM yet. Clinical practice of TCM psychotherapy is also very limited, without systemic theories. According to statistics, there are more than 160 terms of TCM psychotherapy found in Chinese literatures since 1949, which lacks a systemic theory, including working therapy, recreational therapy, exposure therapy of calming, acquisition therapy, five elements therapy, five tone music therapy, five emotions therapy, evil-expelling therapy, Qigong therapy, Qigong-guiding therapy, Qigong-breathing therapy, shocking to calm therapy, panicking therapy, thinking therapy, to treat cheating with deception, to treat malingering with deception, overcoming emotions, mind therapy, calligraphy therapy, persuading therapy, enlightening, heart therapy, psychosomatic transferring therapy, mind-guiding therapy, mental guiding therapy, scheme therapy, arts therapy, persuasion therapy, comforting therapy, demonstration therapy, dream therapy, dream analysis therapy, calming therapy, abreacting therapy, abstinence therapy, training psychotherapy, aversion response therapy, aversion reflex therapy, aversion therapy, environmental therapy, muscle training, natural therapy, farm work therapy, behavioral therapy, behavioral correction therapy, behavioral corrective therapy behavioral guidance therapy, behavioral inducement, behavioral satisfaction therapy, repression therapy, repression and reasoning therapy, joke therapy, drama therapy, guidance therapy, spitting therapy, conspiracy therapy, concentration therapy, fantasy therapy, action and position therapy, rapid stimulation therapy, speech therapy, fraud therapy, extreme therapy, extreme emotion therapy, alcohol therapy, cold water punishment therapy, Buddhist therapy, evil avoiding therapy, talking to guide therapy, circumstance therapy, social therapy, fishing therapy, smearing therapy, relaxation therapy, painting therapy, transfer therapy, distraction therapy, pleasing therapy, Zhuyou exorcism, explanation therapy, language therapy, gratification therapy, satisfaction therapy, seasonal therapy, avoidance therapy, thought therapy, concern therapy, music therapy, adaptation therapy, deterrence therapy, arguing therapy, analysis therapy, beans picking therapy, countering feelings, countering emotions, anger therapy, infuriating therapy, persuading and comforting therapy, belief therapy, drug withdrawal therapy, eliminating concerns, intelligence therapy, humiliation therapy, positive emotional therapy, intimidation therapy, fear therapy, health regulation therapy, temperature therapy, mind cultivation therapy, character cultivation therapy, Taoist therapy, eliminating concerns and pleasing therapy, regulation therapy, counteracting emotions, counteracting conditions, emotional balance therapy, regulating emotions, guiding emotions, relieving the shock, threatening therapy, shocking therapy, qi changing therapy, essence changing therapy, transferring therapy, temperament transforming therapy, placebo therapy, explosion therapy, desensitization therapy, lying therapy, satisfying therapy, gratifying therapy, joy therapy, happiness therapy, revealing therapy, grief therapy, punishing therapy, dream interpretation, pleasurable therapy, weaving therapy, exercising therapy, meditating therapy, education therapy, suggestion therapy, suggestion and guidance therapy, suggestion and disabusing therapy, imagination therapy, anxiety relief therapy, dance therapy, sleep therapy, psychoanalytic therapy, model therapy, imitation therapy, meditation therapy, mind tranquilizing therapy, encouragement therapy, irritating therapy, irritating to purge poison, impulsion therapy, mind emptying therapy, mind emptying and remaining silent therapy.

There are abundant psychological thoughts and techniques of psychotherapy in TCM, but it is very important to choose a proper entrance to explore as there is a tremendous amount of TCM classics. The reason why TCM doctors could cure diseases is that they had reasonable plans, which is contained in medical cases for thousands of years, and thus medical cases are important carriers of TCM psychology. Compared to some subtle and profound theories of TCM psychology, the ancient medical cases about psychotherapy are more concrete and vivid, which bears fascinating wisdom and insights from the ancients. In view of this, we summarize the psychological cases of doctors as far back from the Warring States Period to the Qing Dynasty, and come to the following conclusions of TCM approaches to psychotherapy.

Counteracting emotions, persuasion therapy, suggestion and distraction, satisfaction therapy, to transform temperament, impulsion therapy, to treat malingering with deception, character cultivation (to restore physical and mental health, to erase concerns, to empty the mind, to practice Qigong and Daoyin), drama therapy, scheme therapy (confusion therapy), and dream interpretation are TCM terms from classics, while motivational enhancement therapy, behavioral therapy, and cognitive behavioral therapy are terms of modern psychology.

8.1 Counteracting emotions

Counteracting emotions is a unique psychotherapy in China, which can be firstly found in the *The Inner Canon of the Yellow Emperor* (*Huáng Dì Nèi Jīng*, 黄帝内经) (*hereinafter, Yellow Emperor's Inner Classic*). In a narrow sense, counteracting emotions refers to deliberately using one emotion (appearing later) to control and relieve the symptoms caused by another emotion (appearing before) according to the theory of five elements, so as to cure disease, also known as overcoming emotions.

In a broad sense, counteracting emotions refers to intentionally using one or more emotional triggers to restrict and eliminate mental disorders, so as to treat the psychosomatic illness caused by emotions, according to TCM theories of yin-yang and five elements.

Emotions could not only lead to but also cure diseases. *The Inner Canon of the Yellow Emperor* recognizes mental health and physical health can influence each other physiologically and pathologically and so can different emotions. Therefore, it subtly creates the unique therapy of counteracting emotions, based on the principle of "counteracting." Proper use of emotional therapies can adjust yin and yang, qi and blood, so that the body can restore balance and coordination, curing diseases. *Basic Questions* (*Sù Wèn*, 素问) · *Comprehensive Discourse on Phenomena Corresponding to Yin and Yang* and *Basic Questions* (*Sù Wèn*, 素问) · *Comprehensive Discourse on the Progression of the Five Periods* in *The Inner Canon of the Yellow Emperor* both pointed out that "anger harms the liver; sadness dominates anger; joy harms the heart; fear dominates joy; pensiveness harms the spleen; anger dominates pensiveness; anxiety harms the lung; joy dominates anxiety; fear harms the kidneys; pensiveness dominates fear."

When treating diseases through overcoming emotions, attention should be paid to indications. Generally speaking, emotional therapies can be practiced in diseases with mental disorders as the major illness, but without severe physical health problems. At the same time, attention must be paid to the degree of emotional stimulation. That is to say, therapeutic emotional triggers have to be stronger than emotional factors causing disease. Patients can receive sudden and powerful stimulation if they are physically or psychologically strong. Patients, who are physically or psychologically weak, could constantly receive gradually increased stimulation. In short, emotional triggers to cure disease have to overcome emotional factors causing diseases, otherwise it might fail to take effect. But it must be noted that the degree of stimulation shall not exceed what patients can bear, to avoid causing other emotional disorders.

8.2 Persuasion therapy

Persuasion therapy, as an important form of TCM psychotherapy, has been practiced by doctors consciously or unconsciously from ancient times to the present, benefiting a wide range of health issues.

Persuasion therapy is to eliminate psychological factors causing disease and regulate negative emotions through communications, considering health conditions, psychological states and emotional disorders of patients.

Persuasion therapy includes pleasing and enlightening. Pleasing is to make patients aware of the emotional problems in themselves through persuading and communicating, so that they would actively regulate emotions by themselves, feel eased and then get their emotional illness relieved. Enlightening is to release doubts in patients' mind through the ways such as talking and reasoning, in order to relieve stress and restore mental health.

During persuading, communication skills can be used to build trust with patients in order to find out proper psychotherapy based on their personalities and individual disorders, so that therapies can take effect, pleasing and enlightening patients. *Basic Questions (Sù Wèn, 素问) · Discourse on Moving the Essence and Changing the Qi* reads "Close the door and shut the windows, keep close to patients, repeatedly inquire about feelings, adapt treatment to their sentiments. If one gets a hold of the spirit, the patient will prosper; if the spirit is lost, the patient perishes." Therefore, physicians have to build trust with patients through careful wording and encouragement in a quiet environment, who must have great compassion, serious attitude, and sincere enthusiasm. Then they can make diagnoses when patients tell them about true feelings. The process of speaking out can also help patients to relieve stress and anxiety.

Persuasion should be practiced accordingly based on specific psychological states and individual characteristics of patients. For example, it is said in *The Divine Pivot (Líng Shū, 灵枢) · The Transmissions from the Teachers* that "And further, kings, dukes, and eminent personalities, persons eating bloody meat, they are arrogant, they follow only their own desires, and they look down upon the common people. Hence it is impossible to approach them with dietary prohibitions. If one were to prohibit them something, this would be against their mind. If one were to follow their desires, this would aggravate their disease. To ease their condition, how can this be done? To cure them, what is to be done first? Qi Bo: The intrinsic nature of humans is such: there is no one who does not abhor death and enjoys life. Inform them of what will destroy them. Tell them what will be good for them. Guide them to what will ease their condition. Open their minds to everything that will bring suffering. Even if these are people who do not follow the WAY, why should they not listen?"

This discourse covers four aspects. Firstly, "inform them of what will destroy them" is pointing out the harm of disease to make patients become aware of and understand the disease. Secondly, "tell them what will be good for them" is pointing out that patients can restore health if they follow the advice from doctors properly and timely, so as to boost their confidence in conquering diseases. Thirdly, "guide them to what will ease their condition" is informing patients of what to do and explaining planned treatments to them. Fourthly, "open their minds to everything that will bring suffering" is trying to regulate mental and physical conditions of patients through persuading, explaining, encouraging, comforting, promising and so on.

8.3 Suggestion and distraction

Basic Questions (*Sù Wèn*, 素问) · *Discourse on Regulating the Conduits* reads that "Press and rub affected areas continuously, show needles to patients and tell them: 'I shall insert it deeply.' Once needles approach, they will undergo a change; the essence qi will hide itself internally. The evil qi will disperse in disorder." That is to say, physicians should repeatedly practice pressing and rubbing at the location on patients, where they are going to practice acupuncture, and show needles to the patients, speaking out that the needles will go deeply into body. Then, patients would be concentrated, hiding the essence qi internally, as well as dispersing the evil qi in disorder, so as to improve the effectiveness of acupuncture. That discourse might be the oldest record about suggestion therapy. *The Divine Pivot* (*Líng Shū*, 灵枢) · *To Consider the Spirit as the Foundation* also reads that "All norms of piercing require one to first of all consider the spirit as the foundation." The key for acupuncture to take effect is to receive qi, which relies on the mental condition of patients. Regulating the psychological state of patients with speech and action can help them to receive qi so as to improve the effects of acupuncture.

Suggestion and distraction are to implicitly and indirectly change the psychological state of patients and guide them to follow medical advice from physicians unconsciously. Suggestion and distraction also refer to making patients have faith to change emotions and behaviors. Some physicians also analyze the essence of feelings by language and other means to erase the doubts that patients have, so as to treat diseases caused by emotional factors. That is mostly indicated in patients with hallucinations and depression caused by paranoia.

Suggestion and distraction treat patients through turning their attention away, by means of language or certain objects. Through language, patients can be implicitly and subtly informed of medical knowledge and diseases, which would eliminate negative psychological factors and build confidence to fight against disease, so as to regulate emotions. The language includes speech and behavior. Facial expressions, actions, gestures, placebo and others can be combined flexibly to have more satisfying therapeutic effects. The objects can be drugs and things associated with certain situations, for patients to alleviate psychological suffering. Physicians must identify illness properly and then perform a careful intervention, otherwise it is difficult for therapies to take effect when patients notice the intentions of doctors.

It should be noted that suggestion can be positive or negative. Positive suggestion is often used in medical treatments, while suggestion can cause negative results if performed inappropriately. Therefore, suggestion therapy must be practiced cautiously and flexibly according to the specific psychological conditions of patients. Physicians must be authoritative and influential, qualified with strong analytical reasoning skills and good command of sociology and physiology, so that the suggestion they make can be more positive, stable, lasting and subtle. Suggestion therapy suits malleable patients lack of education better.

8.4 Satisfaction therapy

The Divine Pivot (Líng Shū, 灵枢) · The Transmissions from the Teachers reads "Such an ordering has never succeeded where there is movement contrary to the norms. Now, it is only through a movement in accordance with the norms that a cure is possible... One should see to it that one acts in accordance with the expectations of all the people, the entire population." Besides, "food cravings and sexual desire are basic human instincts," and "it is the human nature to eat when hunger, to warm when cold, to rest when tired, to chase after the good and avoid the bad, which is the same for emperors." To accept inner emotions, patients can have their desires satisfied, which would bring them psychosomatic benefits.

Satisfaction therapy is to release negative psychological factors through meeting the needs of patients mentally and physically, which is indicated in patients failing to go after their wills.

As humans, it is natural to have desires no matter they are good or bad. Physiological and psychological needs are inherent and objective. Whether those needs can be met or not would directly affect emotions and behaviors. It may cause physical and mental health problems if basic desires cannot be satisfied. Persuasion and restraint can hardly end the suffering of patients. "Targeting at the root cause when treating disease" implies that only when basic desires are satisfied can health be recovered. Zhang Jiebin said, "treatments are hard to take effect if concerns causing diseases cannot be erased, going against the will of patients." Simply persuading and transforming temperament can hardly end the suffering of patients or solve mental problems if their reasonable and normal basic desires cannot be satisfied. *The Divine Pivot (Líng Shū,* 灵枢*) · The Transmissions from the Teachers* reads that "one should see to it that one acts in accordance with the expectations of all the people, the entire population," so *Basic Questions (Sù Wèn,* 素问*) · Discourse on Moving the Essence and Changing the Qi* reads that "adapt treatment to their sentiments." Only when basic desires are satisfied, can mental health be restored. In addition to meeting needs, satisfaction therapy also refers to avoiding negative persons and events, which is to protect patients from negative emotional triggers.

Chen Shiduo said "Doctors being obedient to the wishes of patients, patients would accept and benefit from satisfaction therapy. Patients may not listen to doctors and thus refuse to follow advice if they feel offended. So, in ancient times, some patients were asked if they eat dragonflies and butterflies, and they would be catered if saying yes." When patients make unreasonable requests that are hard to be realized, we can try to meet their needs as far as possible if the wishes of patients would not do harm to themselves or others, while if they ask for too much, multiple therapies can be combined, such as comfort, persuasion, aversion, cognitive reframing, etc.

8.5   To transform temperament

Supplement to 'Classified Case Records of Famous Physicians' (Xù Míng Yī Lèi Àn, 续名医 类案*)* reads "to handle frustration has to distract the mind" and "pleasure can remove negative emotions." *History of the Northern Dynasties (Běi Shǐ,* 北史*) · Biography of Cui Guang* advocates that "to have fun through music and books by rivers and lakes helps to relax and restore mental health." Wu Shiji clearly put forward in *Rhymed Discourse on External Remedies (Lǐ Yuè Pián Wén,* 理瀹骈文*)*, that "medications cannot solve emotional problems," so "it would be better to read books and listen to music for regulating seven emotions, rather than taking medicine." However, "emotional regulation skills are supposed to be flexible, in which resorting to flowers and music are just ordinary, so experts in this field must explore further."

To transform temperament actually is to distract attention. Through distraction, the concerns of patients would be eased so as to regulate mental disorders caused by emotions. Activities such as learning and talking can help to ease concerns, reframe thoughts, regulate emotions, break unhealthy habits and develop a good personality.

The events and psychological factors, leading to psychosomatic disorders, can repeatedly upset patients worsening illness, which would establish a vicious circle and prevent recovery. To transform temperament through distraction can divert attention from negative thoughts, so as to manage emotional triggers, just as Wei Zhixiu said "pleasure can remove negative emotions."

This therapy is indicated in patients paying too much attention to their problems, which prevents their recovery. It is also indicated in patients worrying too much about certain parts of their body, which leads to abnormal involuntary movements. Besides, it can be used to regulate disorders caused by excessive preoccupation.

To transform temperament is not to suppress emotions or deny personalities, but to divert attentions so as to remove negative emotional factors and improve personalities. So, this therapy has a wide range of applications with various techniques. All in all, it should be practiced flexibly, considering subjective and objective factors such as specific situations, psychological states, interests, surroundings, conditions, etc.

8.6   Impulsion therapy

Ancient doctors found in clinical practice that patients with extreme impulsions often had conducts beyond physical limits, normally impossible to happen, which bore predictable functions.

Impulsion therapy is to arouse impulsions and make use of the expected extreme conducts, so as to regulate physical health conditions.

It is difficult to practice impulsion therapy, which tends to be misunderstood by patients. If practiced inappropriately, the therapy can do harm to patients, making them feel humiliated, causing a series of serious consequences. Therefore, it should be only taken as a last resort.

8.7   To treat malingering with deception

Malingering is the feigning of illness, of which pulse patterns and treatments were clearly recorded in *The Pulse Classic* (*Mài Jīng*, 脉经). Zhang Jingyue later proposed that "to deceive patients with their own deception would reveal the true and cure malingerers."

To treat malingering with deception is to pay patients with their own coins. In other words, doctors assess the malingering and then practice deception therapies to force malingerers back to normal, making use of their weakness.

Assessment of malingering is important before treating malingering with deception. There are various motives behind malingering, leading to different manifestations, which brings a lot of difficulties to doctors. Doctors shall not rush to make a diagnosis if the pulse of patients does not match the symptoms of malingering. Diagnoses must be made according to pulse conditions, pathogenesis, disease course, emotional responses, and physical health conditions. Modern laboratory technologies can be resorted to when necessary. Only when all the above elements are taken into consideration and the diagnosis of malingering is ascertained can corresponding treatments be given.

During treatment, doctors should let patients know through appropriate words and actions that their malingering has been detected. Then, targeting at the weakness of patients, therapies can be practiced accordingly. Chances should be given to patients who tend to retreat from malingering. Doctors can threaten those who fear being exposed that they will be exposed, and those who refuse to receive injury treatments that injury therapies will be practiced. But the prerequisite is that family members and people around patients have to cooperate with doctors, who shall not hurt the self-esteem of patients or humiliate them, to avoid new psychological disorders.

Differences between hypochondriasis and malingering must be identified during clinical practice. Malingerers have subjective motives for personal gain, while hypochondriasis does not have such motives, characterized by excessive preoccupation with their health conditions.

8.8 Character cultivation

Mind cultivation derives from "to put family in order has to cultivate oneself first" in *Book of Rites* (*Lǐ Jì*, 礼记) · *The Great Learning*, which is to mold temperament and improve personality. Mind cultivation is one of the eight items of Confucian education. Nature cultivation derives from "to preserve one's mental constitution, and nourish one's nature, is the way to serve Heaven" in The *Works of Mencius* (*Mèng Zǐ*, 孟子) · *Jin Xin I*, that is to restore physical and mental health and to cultivate moral character. Character cultivation is a Taoist practice to stay in a quiet space alone and empty the mind. Character cultivation also refers to life cultivation, keeping healthy to extend lifespan.

Character cultivation is a terminology of Confucianism, which refers to the maintenance of body and mind, but it has a specific meaning in TCM psychology, referring to psychosomatic cultivation.

Explanations of Words in Classics (*Jīng Jí Zuǎn Gǔ*, 经籍纂诂) reads that "human natures are inborn characteristics," which are inherent but can also be molded, including temperament and character traits. The natures determine emotional tendencies of an individual. People of different personalities are vulnerable to different emotional triggers, so that they would have different psychological disorders. Those who are good at character cultivation can balance emotions well, keeping yin and yang at peace, so as to stay healthy.

So, character cultivation is to educate oneself, establish a healthy lifestyle, build good habits, improve personality, enhance social adaptation skills, and maintain a balanced physical and mental condition.

Those who are good at character cultivation can balance emotions well, keeping yin and yang at peace, so as to stay healthy. So, it is important to regulate psychosomatic disorders and balance emotions, which helps to eliminate negative emotions and adjust physical and mental conditions. In particular, character cultivation can help patients to prevent psychosomatic diseases, which targets at the very root of cause.

8.9 Drama therapy

Holism of TCM implies that diseases are closely related to environments. Therefore, for patients with psychosomatic disorders, it is not enough to adjust physical and mental conditions. Drama therapy should be used to change the surroundings for patients.

Drama therapy is to change the unfavorable surroundings preventing recovery and avoid constant stimulation by negative psychological triggers.

Living environments are both natural and social. The social environments can be as large as the whole society and as small as a family and specific living condition. Drama therapy is highly targeted at eliminating the emotional triggers leading to psychological disorders and preventing recovery.

It should be noted that when people cannot adapt themselves to the surroundings well, most of them would consciously or unconsciously make efforts to improve the environment or adjust themselves. In that process, initiative is very important. Drama therapy is to artificially prevent negative emotional triggers and gratify patients. Therefore, patients would fail to adapt themselves to the surroundings once they come to adverse environments. Character cultivation therapy can help improve adaptability to relieve stress.

8.10 Scheme therapy (Confusion therapy)

Confusion therapy derives from a military science to "make a feint to the east but attack in the west" in *Comprehensive Statutes* (*Tōng Diǎn*, 通典) · *Military Affairs Six*, deceiving your opponent.

Ancient physicians learned scheme therapy from military strategists, which is to give a sudden treatment to patients in relaxation after diverting their attentions when they cannot normally cooperate with doctors. The method must "be cunning to manipulate thoughts, which should not be indicated in people who have no resources."

Before practicing scheme therapy, doctors have to get familiar with the personality traits of patients, so as to make an accurate diagnosis and prognosis, and then provide with a proper treatment plan accordingly. It must be avoided to blindly use scheme therapy without adequate preparations.

To practice scheme therapy, doctors must take comprehensive advantage of sociology, demonstrating that TCM requires skills in addition to technologies. Traditional Chinese emotional (psychological) therapies are promising in the future of medicine. Emotional (psychological) therapies used to be and will continue to be an advantage of TCM. However, in modern society, emphasis on the protection of privacy and human rights of patients makes it hard to use some extreme therapies (such as cheating, intimidating, infuriating and seducing). Furthermore, people gradually lose interest in the application of and the in-depth research on emotional therapies, due to low economic benefits, high risks and difficulties in quantitative evaluation of therapeutic effects. It is significant to modify and improve those extreme therapies so that they become more applicable.

8.11 Dream interpretation

Preoccupation with dreams can cause diseases. Dream Interpretation is to analyze the dreams patients had and eliminate misunderstandings of dreams based on their psychogenic disorders.

China was the first country to conduct study on dreams. Ancient people believed that dreams were closely related to future weal and woe, so they were keen on interpreting dreams. They often used dreams to predict good or ill luck. There is a book *The Duke of Zhou's Explanation of Dreams* (*Zhōu Gōng Jiě Mèng*, 周公解梦) written in the name of the Duke of Zhou, which lists objects and events of dream and explains their meanings associated with actual lives.

Instead of rigidly adhering to *The Duke of Zhou's Explanation of Dreams* (*Zhōu Gōng Jiě Mèng*, 周公解梦), medical experts in previous dynasties made reasonable interpretation of dreams for patients based on collected information of family backgrounds, social status and health conditions through inspection, listening and smelling, inquiring and palpation, so that they could achieve expected therapeutic effects.

Dreams as a phenomenon of life, with infinite mysteries, have been appealing to human for thousands of years, but its mechanism cannot be fully explained yet. Modern studies reveal that the events and scenes in a dream come from memories, including visual, audio, tactile, and emotional memories. So, dreams are almost constructed out of memories.

The Chinese nation promotes self-examination and has faith in destiny, so people often believe that dreams can predict good or ill luck and thus pay close attention to dreams. *The Duke of Zhou's Explanation of Dreams* (*Zhōu Gōng Jiě Mèng*, 周公解梦) is a collection of dreams, usually considered ridiculous due to rigid adherence by ignoring individual differences although it records the exploration of dreams by ancient people.

Past generations of physicians were normally well-educated, not blinded by previous thoughts. Through clinical practice for a long period of time, it is found that dreams consist of physiological and psychological aspects. Therefore, to eliminate misunderstandings of dreams requires not only dealing with physical health problems but also regulating emotions, taking both physical and mental health problems into consideration.

Dream interpretation is generally divided into direct interpretation and indirect interpretation. Direct interpretation of dreams is completely made by doctors, conducting analysis to erase doubts and get rid of anxiety in patients. Indirect dream interpretation refers to patients restructuring the understanding of dreams under guidance of a doctor, so as to regulate emotions.

Dreams consist of physiological and psychological aspects, but the mechanism cannot be fully explained yet. Therefore, dream interpretation must be used cautiously in clinical practice. Before dream interpretation, physical and mental health conditions of patients must be fully understood and their desires could be assessed if necessary. Doctors must build trust with patients and completely comprehend the misunderstandings of dreams by patients so that cognitive restructuring can be effective to get rid of doubts.

8.12 Motivational Enhancement Therapy

Motivational enhancement therapy is a therapy of self-regulation for patients to handle psychosomatic diseases by themselves.

Motivational enhancement therapy is for patients to actively divert attention from themselves to other objects or activities so as to change mind and balance emotions, indicated in mental disorders caused by emotions.

The therapy can only be used for people with proper mental competence, who can conduct self-examination appropriately, but not for malleable people lack of education or self-knowledge.

8.13 Behavioral Therapy

The Inner Canon of the Yellow Emperor (*Huáng Dì Nèi Jīng*, 黄帝内经) reads that "internal conditions are to be displayed externally." If a person has disease internally, it is definitely reflected externally. Similarly, inner temperament and mental state can be projected on behaviors. Therefore, cognitive and emotional states can be adjusted by changing behaviors over time.

Behavioral therapy is an achievement in experimental psychology, which helps patients change behaviors for healing. Although TCM has no such term as behavioral therapy, it regards mental disorders and physical symptoms as abnormal behaviors, which believes that behaviors can be adjusted and changed to restore health through learning.

TCM behavioral therapies are varied to regulate emotions, with the commonly seen methods including acquisition therapy (desensitization therapy), corrective therapy, behavior inducement, behavioral satisfaction, tension therapy, etc.

Acquisition therapy is similar to desensitization therapy. That is to find out causes of fear first and gradually expose patients to emotional triggers increasingly, aiming to build immunity to the triggers, getting rid of fear, relieving stress and finally restoring physical and mental health.

Corrective therapy is to regulate behaviors by imposing proper punishments, associating symptoms with unpleasant experience.

Behavior inducement refers to guiding patients to get rid of abnormal behaviors.

Behavioral satisfaction is to meet the behavioral needs of patients and remove pathogenic factors.

Tension therapy is to expose patients to circumstances or substances causing intense fear, in order to quickly eliminate misunderstandings of fear and anxiety triggers, and to get rid of subconscious stress.

As a technology of modern medicine, behavioral therapy only has a history of nearly one hundred years, in lack of a cohesive and coherent theoretical support. However, behavioral approaches have been widely used in TCM clinical practice. It should be noted that expediency technique of behavioral satisfaction must be used very carefully, because although such lying is out of goodwill, it will bring negative effects and lead to relapse if used improperly. *Comments on Ancient and Modern Case Records* (*Gǔ Jīn Yī Àn Àn*, 古今医案按) · *Volume Six* · *Notes on Madness* by Yu Zhen reads, "That is why mental illness has to be dealt with mental approaches. Once upon a time, poverty brought a patient suffering. Doctors asked people to grant the patient a fortune, who thus recovered. However, that was only of expediency. Relapse would occur once the truth is suddenly revealed. Therefore, it is better to guide patients to change their mind so as to ultimately prevent relapse." Before practicing tension therapy, patients should be informed of its fundamentals and how it works, especially the suffering they would experience during treatment. Physical and mental examinations should be conducted in advance. Tension therapy is contraindicated in patients with cardiovascular disease, endocrine disease, epilepsy and severe mental illness.

8.14 Cognitive Behavioral Therapy

Cognitive behavioral therapy aims to modify thought patterns of conventional thinking, belief and mindset, in order to help patients to overcome emotional and behavioral disorders. This therapy has evolved from behavior modification and behavioral therapy.

Cognitive behavioral therapy came into being in the late 1970s, but it was recorded in ancient Chinese medical cases long ago.

Classified Case Records of Famous Physicians (*Míng Yī Lèi Àn*, 名医类案) · *Volume Eight · Mental Disorder of Madness* reads that Kuang Ziyuan "had no chance to go back to hometown during working as an academician for more than 10 years, and thus felt frustrated and disoriented at the onset of mental illness, sometimes being delirious, but back to normal when the illness disappeared." Kwang was an official, working far away from home, who often felt dazed with mental and emotional disorders. An old monk in Zhenkong temple, who achieved the WAY, firstly pointed out directly that the mental disorder of Kuang "began at concerns, worsen by delusions." Then, knowing Kuang was an academician, he educated Kuang by analyzing the harm of "delusions from the past, at present and in the future." Kuang also learned about "exogenous and endogenous desires" and the harm of "overstress," and was thus "aware of his wrong and inappropriate delusions." Kuang followed advise from the monk to remove delusions and change behaviors "to practice staying in a room alone and emptying the mind, and mental health was restored a month later." The treatment advised by the old monk coincides with cognitive behavioral therapy in modern psychology.

"Unity of knowledge and action" is the essence of traditional Chinese culture, so TCM attaches great importance to harmony between mind and body. It is believed that cognition is the basis of behaviors and emotions, so behavioral and emotional disorders are closely related to cognitive disorders. It is true that some psychosomatic symptoms can be alleviated or eliminated by correcting external abnormal behaviors, but therapeutic effects will not be lasting and relapse will occur frequently without cognitive regulation. TCM advocates guiding patients to get rid of wrong mindsets, and improve their adaptability, so as to help them overcome emotional and behavioral disorders and restore physical and mental health. Firstly, in clinical practice, patients should be helped to understand the relationship between their wrong mindsets and emotional and behavioral disorders. Secondly, it is necessary to make in-depth analyses of the thoughts that patients have, and help them distinguish healthy mentalities from harmful ones, so as to improve adaptability. It is also essential to help patients master some skills to strengthen adaptability, including how to develop a new mindset.

LECTURE 9

Harmony in Diversity

Stagnation Syndrome in TCM vs Depression in Western Medicine

LECTURER: WANG QINGQI, WANG ZHEN

Introduction to the speaker:

Wang Qingqi is a tenured professor in Shanghai University of Traditional Chinese Medicine, with the title of Shanghai Famous TCM Doctor. Entitled to special government allowances from the State Council in China, he is an academic experience inheritance instructor of national outstanding TCM experts, who has trained 40 students including PhD students, post-doctoral fellows and academic inheritors. He is also an editor-in-chief of TCM for *Chinese Dictionary of Etymology* (*Ci Hai*, 辞海). Prof. Wang has been engaged in the practice of TCM internal medicine (involving digestive diseases and psychosomatic disorders) and in teaching *The Inner Canon of the Yellow Emperor* (*Huáng Dì Nèi Jìng*, 黄帝内经) for over 50 years. He has been an editor-in-chief and an associate editor-in-chief for more than 50 academic books. He won the first prize of Shanghai TCM Science and Technology Awards and the second prize of China Association of Chinese Medicine Science and Technology Award. Besides, he is the host of TCM Psychology Master Studio funded by Shanghai Municipal Education Commission.

Wang Zhen, PhD., physician-in-chief, postdoctoral supervisor, is a vice president of Shanghai Mental Health Center affiliated to Shanghai Jiao Tong University School of Medicine. He is a member of CBT coordination group in Society of Psychiatry of Chinese Medical Association, and the vice president of Research League of Obsessive-

Compulsive Disorder in Research Branch of Basic and Clinical Psychiatry of China Neuroscience Society. Prof. Wang has been engaged in researches on clinical practice and disease mechanism of obsessive-compulsive disorder, anxiety disorders, emotional and psychological trauma, as well as common emotional problems.

Wang Qingqi: For more than 10 years, I have been interested in depression because of two reasons. One is that there are many incisive insights into psychosomatic disorders in a TCM classic *The Inner Canon of the Yellow Emperor* (*Huáng Dì Nèi Jīng*, 黄帝内经) written more than 2500 years ago, which is the oldest book with documentation of psychological disorders and very intriguing to me. The other is that I have found TCM can benefit many patients with commonly seen spleen and stomach problems, which can be obviously improved in several months after treatment. And among the patients who did not achieve satisfying therapeutic effects, many of them actually had mental disorders to different extents, such as depression and anxiety. That set me thinking. Why was that so? After reading literature of TCM and Western medicine, I realized mental disorders including depression and anxiety were primary reasons behind difficulties in treating spleen and stomach problems. Nowadays, more and more doctors in digestive system department and the department of psychiatry pay attention to the relation between mental factors and diseases of digestive system. Some hospitals have already established specialty clinics for digestive diseases affected by mental disorders. I compared the documentation of stagnation syndrome in TCM literature with depression and anxiety in modern medicine. Based on that, I would like to share my clinical experiences and conclusions.

9.1 *"Stagnation" and "Stagnation Syndrome"*

9.1.1 *The Concept of "Stagnation"*

In TCM, depression is called stagnation syndrome. 郁 (*yù*, stagnation) in Chinese has a broad connotation, involving constraint and blockage. According to plenty of medical literature comparing stagnation, constraint and retention in TCM, 郁 (*yù*, stagnation) in Chinese mainly has two connotations. One refers to disease mechanism in TCM, corresponding to pathomechanism in Western medicine, which reveals a pathological condition where qi and blood are blocked so that zang-fu organs can not work properly. The other refers to a concept of disease, denoting that stagnation syndrome is mainly characterized by stagnant qi movement resulting from depressed moods. There are overlaps and and differences between these two explanations, with one putting emphasis on pathomechanism and the other on the concept. Besides, 郁 (*yù*, stagnation) can have other implications, so the exact meaning it refers to should be determined in specific contexts. Anyway, disease with pathomechanism of depression and stagnation is named stagnation syndrome in TCM.

The Inner Canon of the Yellow Emperor: Basic Questions (Huáng Dì Nèi Jīng Sù Wèn, 黄帝内经素问) · *Comprehensive Discourse on The Policies and Arrangements of The Six Principal Qi* mentions stagnation, involving the stagnation in qi movement of five periods. Qi movement refers to climate and weather influenced by qi moving. TCM uses six elements to describe physical phenomena of the atmosphere in the nature, including wind, cold, summerheat, dampness, dryness, fire. In the normal state, the six elements are named "six qi," illustrating the features of atmosphere, weather and climate. In the summer, heat qi dominates, leading to hot weather with hot fire qi. Wind dominates the spring, so there is wind qi. In late summer, rain brings dampness qi. Therefore, qi mentioned here refers to climatic phenomena caused by qi moving and transforming.

People in ancient China used the theory of five elements, namely, metal, wood, water, fire, earth, to explain the phenomena resulting from qi transforming. Corresponding to the five elements, six qi turns into the five of cold, summerheat, dryness, dampness and wind. Then, for example, wind pertains to wood; cold pertains to water; dryness pertains to metal; heat and summerheat pertains to fire. The six qi have generating and restraining relationships among each other, and so have the five elements. The generating order is wood, fire, earth, metal and water; while the restraining order is wood, earth, water, fire and metal. That is to say, wood generates fire; fire generates earth; earth generates metal; metal generates water; water generates wood; wood restrains earth; earth restrains water; water restrains fire; fire restrains metal; metal restrains wood. It demonstrates such a relationship of generating and restraining among the five elements in the nature. It embodies ancient Chinese philosophy, leading TCM to explain pathogenesis accordingly.

For instance, wood stands for wind and earth stands for dampness. If wind qi gets stronger, wood will thrive to restrain earth. In the nature, the earth getting wet after raining, it would become dry even without the sun if there is strong wind, which is called wood overwhelming earth. An old Chinese saying that "anything is restrained by something" implies generating and restraining relationships among things. Thus, stagnation denotes an abnormal phenomenon. When such stagnation gets worse, it might fight back.

There are "five stagnations" regarding qi movement and transformation, specifically earth stagnation, wood stagnation, metal stagnation, fire stagnation, and water stagnation. Earth stagnation results from restraint by wood qi; wood stagnation results from restraint by metal qi, namely dry qi; metal stagnation results from restraint by fire, and so on and so forth. These also reveal a Chinese way of thinking to understand climatic change in the nature with the rules of generating and restraining.

Under the circumstances of five stagnations, abnormal climatic phenomena will lead to epidemics or frequently occurring diseases. For example, earth stagnation implies great dampness, and too much dampness can cause diseases including arthritis, edema, and even gastrointestinal diseases. When the weather is wet, people may have poor appetite. High pressure in the air inhibits the digestive function of the spleen and the stomach so that people feel full in the abdomen. Therefore, extra dampness in the environment can weaken transporting and transforming activities in the spleen and the stomach, thus causing poor appetite. That is why TCM fortifies the spleen to remove dampness. Then, how can we know if a disease is caused by dampness? There are two ways to identify. One is to observe climatic change. The other is to determine based on tongue coating, pulse taking, and symptoms corresponding to dampness encumbering the stomach and spleen.

Specifically speaking, stagnation denotes a phenomenon of change in weather or climate.

9.1.2 Stagnation in a broad sense

Stagnation in a broad sense involves physiology and pathology, including external pathogens and internal damage. TCM classifies causes of disease into three categories. The first one is external pathogens, referring to abnormal climatic change invading human body. The second one is internal damage, referring to emotional change, especially serious mental trauma and disease caused by social pressure. The third is the in-between, such as improper diet, and fatigue due to overexertion. Those three categories of causes of disease can lead to stagnation in qi and blood, as in the stagnation in a broad sense.

Medical expert Zhu Danxi in Yuan dynasty said disease would not occur when qi and blood maintain harmony, but any illness could happen once there is stagnation. TCM believes the human body consists of qi and blood, with qi and blood unceasingly operating inside the human body to maintain life. How can one stay alive and energetic? Qi and blood bring us vitality to fight against disease, and that is why "disease would not occur when qi and blood maintain harmony." In other words, qi and blood operating regularly inside the body help you stay healthy. "Any illness could happen once there is stagnation." That is to say, internal damage and external pathogens, inhibiting qi and blood from operating regularly, are causes of disease providing environments for disease to occur. Therefore, "human disease mostly arises from stagnation." From this perspective, all the causes of disease, no matter internal or external, can disturb qi and blood, thus leading to stagnation in a broad sense. For example, if coronary arteries are over 75% obstructed, agina could occur, implying "operating successfully but not regularly." If they are 100% obstructed, myocardial infarction would occur, implying "failure to operate." "Operating successfully but not regularly" causes disease, while "failure to operate" threatens life. Therefore, TCM believes that stagnation is the origin of all diseases and all diseases involve qi and blood stagnation.

Specifically, the sayings are concerned with depression. For example, depression can be caused by emotional disorders and innate character flaws. In addition, other diseases caused by depression, such as heart disease, hypertension, diabetes and nervous system disorders, all belong to psychosomatic disorders. Psychosomatic disorders refer to physical illnesses caused by mental factors, including hypertension, coronary artery disease, neurodermatitis, asthma, rheumatic arthritis, and rheumatoid arthritis. Today, cancers are also included in psychosomatic disorders. Scleroderma and ankylosing spondylitis are concomitant symptoms of depression. Therefore, stagnation syndrome in a broad sense in TCM, covers more than that of functional disorders in a limited sense, involving various diseases instead of climatic factors.

1) *Comprehensive Medicine According to Master Zhang* (*Zhāng Shì Yī Tōng*, 张氏医通) in Qing dynasty records the stagnation syndrome caused by seven emotions. The stagnation syndrome of seven emotions is also named internal stagnation, because emotions are internal and emotional stagnation can lead to illness. For example, "anger without expression" is to suppress anger inside the body and cause stagnation of qi and blood in zang-fu organs, leading to physical illness, which is also named "anger stagnation." Likewise, sorrow stagnation refers to illness caused by suppressed sorrow. Other types of stagnation syndrome also have such similar pathogenesis. In clinic, stagnation syndrome of seven emotions is a type of depression caused by emotional suppression.

2) *Comprehensive Medicine According to Master Zhang* (*Zhāng Shì Yī Tōng*, 张氏医通) in Qing dynasty also records the stagnation syndrome caused by six qi, namely wind, cold, summerheat, dampness, dryness, and fire. For example, the wet weather with low air pressure may lead to poor appetite, heavy limbs, and fatigue among people with spleen and stomach illness. That is called "dampness stagnation" because dampness in the nature invades the spleen and stomach. TCM treats it by resolving dampness and relieving stagnation.

3) *Teachings of [Zhu] Dan-xi* (*Dān Xī Xīn Fǎ*, 丹溪心法) by Zhu Danxi in Yuan dynasty records six types of stagnation syndrome, including qi stagnation, heat stagnation, phlegm stagnation, dampness stagnation, blood stagnation and food stagnation. They are mainly caused by internal damage, climatic factors and diets. Zhu Danxi invented famous formulas of Liuyu Tang (六郁汤, Decoction for Six Stagnations) and Yueju Wan (越鞠丸, Depression-Resolving Pill) with great therapeutic effects on six stagnation syndromes.

4) *Black Pearl from Red Waters* (*Chì Shuǐ Xuán Zhū*, 赤水玄珠) by Sun Yikui in Ming dynasty records stagnation syndrome of five zang-organs. Five zang-organs are heart, liver, spleen, lung and kidney, with unique physiological functions and dynamic physiological activities, which normally work without stagnation. For example, the heart is an organ in the circulatory system. It has to operate smoothly, otherwise stagnation can cause angina, with a mild symptom of cardiac arrhythmia or a serious symptom of myocardial infarction, revealing "heart stagnation." Liver stagnation happens when negative emotions inhibit liver qi movement, leading to loss of appetite. For example, when a couple take their quarrels to heart, it is regraded as liver qi stagnation in TCM. If they make peace a few days later, then liver stagnation would disappear. If they keep negative emotions for over half a year, it can turn into depression.

The above definitions of depression are made from different perspectives, which belong to stagnation syndrome in a broad sense. They involve opinions of TCM experts in previous generations, taken as important guidelines for TCM clinical syndrome differentiation and treatment, but they are not completely equal to the depression in Western medicine.

9.1.3 Stagnation in a limited sense

Stagnation in a limited sense of TCM is similar to the depression in Western medicine, referring to illness caused by depressed moods and stagnation of qi movement, with symptoms including negative emotions, restlessness, gas pain in the chest, and pain under ribs. But that is not completely equal to the depression in Western medicine. In Western medicine, there are criteria to identify depression, while the notion of stagnation syndrome in TCM is comparatively vague with a broader range of criteria.

9.2 Melancholy and depression

Melancholy refers to an emotion. Modern psychology defines emotions as attitudes to things, temporarily revealing whether there is satisfaction. When people want to buy something, they desire but fail to get, and feel unpleasant. Is that depression? The answer is no. The unpleasant feeling would disappear a few days later or can be relieved when people finally get what they want. The feeling is temporary in the condition of failure to satisfy desires.

Emotions can be classified into positive and negative emotions. Melancholy is negative. No matter they are positive or negative, emotions are based on the experience of satisfaction. As a saying goes, worldviews decide needs and desires, and then needs and desires determine behaviors. Corresponding reactions would occur when needs and desires cannot be catered to. We need to understand melancholy is a negative emotion. Long lasting bouts of negative emotions are considered as a cause of internal damage in TCM. In this regard, TCM and Western medicine share the same opinion.

In Western medicine, depression involves several groups of symptoms, characterized by three key forms of cognitive disorder with enduring low moods, namely negative opinions about self-esteem, environments and the future. Depression is manifested in the following four aspects.

1) Emotional distress. Emotions are different from moods. Moods are temporary, while emotions last longer, being comparatively stable. Symptoms of depression include loss of interest in the surroundings, lack of confidence, worthlessness, hopelessness, helplessness, and loss of motivation. Based on clinical observations, 40% patients have those symptoms.

2) Retarded thinking. Clinical symptoms include less talking, slow speech, and subjective experience of slowness and laboriousness in the flow of thoughts.

3) Decreased energy. Symptoms include slow movements, passiveness, laziness, desire to be idle, avoidance of contact with people, loneliness and social isolation.

4) It could be considered as depression if the above symptoms last for more than half a year without any improvement. Otherwise, it involves depressed mood at the outside but can not be diagnosed as depression.

Apparently, Western medicine and TCM describe causes and manifestations of depression in different ways. TCM explains it in a comparatively general way, lack of proper quantification or clear presentation. In terms of psychiatry, four common depression types are bipolar disorder, persistent depressive disorder, situational depression and depression during menopause, classified based on age, manifestations, causes of disease.

In a limited sense, depression refers to bipolar disorder, also named endogenous depression. People, with a low amount of some biological and chemical substances inside the body (such as serotonin) for a long time, are vulnerable to endogenous depression, also known as major depressive disorder. Clinically, Western medicine usually does not further classify the types of depression because they share the same treatments. In terms of psychiatry, it is necessary to further classify them based on causes of depression because treatments can be different.

WHO statistics show the global incidence of depression is 11%, with approximately 340 million patients. Depression is ranked as the fourth leading cause of disease burden worldwide, following cardiovascular disease, cerebrovascular disease and cancers. There was a report reading that "depression happens when the mind catches cold." But I do not agree because it can be self-healing when you literally catch cold but depression usually cannot be self-healing. Today, there are two main reasons for increasing incidence of depression. Firstly, in the society of market economy, people have to compete for interests. Some people succeed and some fail, who all would encounter mental pressure. If managed improperly, psychological imbalance can lead to mental disorders and even depression. Secondly, even though people live stable and wealthy lives, they are vulnerable to mental disorders if they do not have full spiritual life with lack of common sense on mental health. I read an article titled *The Void* in Shanghai *Liberation Daily*, by a Shanghai writer traveling in the U.S. The article is short but impressive with a sentence that "people lack of nothing are in danger." When people are lack of nothing, they usually have nothing spiritual to chase after. So in fact, they are lack of spiritual support, thus being bored and spiritually empty, which might lead to melancholy. Therefore, it is good when people are lack of something and then they can have something to chase after. For example, if a couple want to buy a car, they would save 2000 yuan every month. They can feel happy because they have a target, so they normally are not vulnarable to depression. However, after they buy a car and a villa and their children grow up and enter college, they might have nothing to chase after and feel empty, which actually could bring melancholy to them.

I met a housewife with a rich family background, but she had insomnia. I asked her why. She said she had nothing to worry about and she was proud she had a villa, a BMW car and her son went to Harvard university. In daily life, she had nothing to do but kept thinking too much. She got insomnia for a long time and it turned out to be melancholy. So, nothing to chase after is a new social phenomenon nowadays. In the past, China was poor. In a certain way, being poor may prevent melancholy because being poor can motivate people to work hard. Therefore, it is a new social problem that idleness can lead to melancholy today.

The most dreadful is not depression itself, but the intention to commit suicide comes after depression among some patients. I am not a psychiatrist but I had some patients with intention to commit suicide. I mainly treat digestive system diseases with TCM, and I find that many patients with digestive disorders usually also have mental disorders. Once I bought a book about the basic and clinical research of digestive system in psychosomatic perspective. It explains from the view of Western medicine and I was inspired. If doctors in departments of digestive diseases do not know how to manage depression and anxiety of patients, the therapeutic effects for digestive disorders would not be satisfying. There are more than 90 million people suffering from depression in China, with more women than men. According to *The Inner Canon of the Yellow Emperor* (*Huáng Dì Nèi Jīng*, 黄帝内经), females are usually with redundant qi in terms of body constitution. The qi refers to pathogenic qi but not healthy original qi. Especially during menopause, women can have insomnia because of trifles, so they easily get upset. It is astonishing that people more than 2500 years ago could conclude females are vulnarable to anger and liver qi stagnation.

9.3 Depression and anxiety disorders

Sometimes, depression is mixed up with anxiety disorders. Based on psychiatry records, the probability of anxiety disorders following depression is 60% and it is reported that 30%-90% of depression can have the complication of anxiety disorders. Normally patients have depression at the beginning and then both depression and anxiety disorders afterwards.

According to psychiatry clinical practice guidelines, if a patient has both depression and anxiety disorders, it should be diagnosed as depression as a priority. There is no such disease named depression or anxiety disorders in TCM, but TCM considers anxiety disorders are based on depression. Then what exactly is an anxiety disorder? An anxiety disorder is a mental illness involving constant and chronic worrying, uneasiness and fear. In my understanding, anxiety is different from fear. Fear is to worry about what has happened, while anxiety is to worry about what has not happened, is going to happen and even will not happen. Groundless worry is a typical manifestation of anxiety disorders, namely worrying about something that acutually does not exist. The incidence of anxiety disorders was 1% to 2% in 1980s, and now is 13%.

Also, normal anxiety is different from anxiety disorders. Normal anxiety is an unpleasant emotion with nervousness, expected based on certain events challenging to manage. For example, an inexperienced doctor may tell patients that atrophic gastritis can lead to precancerous lesions, without further explanation. Generally speaking, the statement is not wrong, but common people could mistake precancerous lesions as cancers and then they get anxious and panic, but in fact cancers have not happened. Actually, the rate of cancer occurrence in patients with atrophic gastritis is only 1%–3%.

Normal anxiety is beneficial and it can help people to get prepared and adjust their behaviors, which is a human instinct to adapt to environmental changes. This is why people usually say "being prepared for the unexpected." For instance, at present TCM competes actively with Western medicine to win over medical markets. If

TCM does not have supportive policies, the mainstream of Western medicine will take over market areas of TCM. By time, it would be hard for TCM to survive. So TCM must get prepared for the unexpected future, which raises normal anxiety and is beneficial to the development of TCM. The normal anxiety is positive and beneficial to health, rather than problem anxiety leading to anxiety disorders. The following is about signs and symptoms of anxiety disorders.

1) Excessive worrying. It refers to being worried about dangerous or bad things that actually are not going to happen, leading to nervousness, fear, hypervigilance, insomnia and irritability. Typically, such diseases as asthma, cardiac neurosis and gastric neurosis involve different levels of anxiety. That is why diseases in the spleen and stomach are related to psychological factors, specifically anxiety.
2) Psychomotor agitation. It involves movements including rubbing hands, stamping feet, walking back and forth, failure to sit still, finger twitching, shaking and tremors, etc.
3) Autonomic hyperactivity. It is manifested by palpitations, rapid breathing, dizziness, dry mouth, profuse sweating, frequent and urgent urination, redness on face, globus sensation, stomach discomfort, diarrhea, sexual dysfunction, etc. Typical signs of autonomic hyperactivity are frequent urination, and irritable bowel syndrome. Abdominal pain and diarrhea are typical symptoms of anxiety disorders. Like depression, anxiety disorders last for more than six months. If relieved in a couple of weeks, it could be regarded as positive normal anxiety. Anxiety disorders may accompany other mental disorders such as depression, schizophrenia, obsessive compulsive disorder, phobia, neurasthenia, etc.

About the differences in depression and anxiety disorders, there are a few key points apart from the above characteristics.

1) Depression is characterized by low mood, while anxiety disorders are characterized by tension and fear.
2) In terms of clinical manifestations, depression is featured by sorrow, helplessness, desperation, guilt and loss of interest, while anxiety disorders are featured by presistent fear and worry.
3) Depression can be accompanied by anxiety disorders, diabetes, cancers, heart diseases, etc. Anxiety disorders can also be accompanied by depression, migraine, heart diseases, functional gastrointestinal disorders, etc. Depression and anxiety disorders can be the cause of each other, with usually depression leading to anxiety disorders. Depression and anxiety disorders can come hand in hand, taking up more than 60% of the overall situation.

4) From the perspective of diagnosis, depression is more concerned about what has happened and the patients feel guilty and sad, thinking the future must be worse than the past. For example, in a class reunion, when people gather together without meeting each other for many years, they would have some pleasant conversations. However, people with depression would say there is no never-ending feast. They always think about things from negative perspectives. People with anxiety disorders are extremely concerned about the future, about the things that are going to happen or the things will not happen, so as to avoid risks.

5) In terms of lifestyle, patients with depression usually keep silent. They can have sleep disorders, poor concentration, retarded thinking, and intention to commit suicide. Patients with anxiety disorders are disturbed by stubborn thinking, restlessness, profuse swearing, hyperventilation, etc., which may interfere with others' lives.

In TCM, according to *The Inner Canon of the Yellow Emperor* (*Huáng Dì Nèi Jīng*, 黄帝内经), patience pertains to yin and restlessness pertains to yang. So based on clinical manifestations, depression belongs to yin syndrome and anxiety disorders belong to yang syndrome, with depression featured by silence, introversion, reluctance to move, and anxiety disorders featured by worry, hyperactivity, and restlessness.

9.4 Causes of depression

9.4.1 The Causes

(1) BODY CONSTITUTION.

In TCM theory of body constitution, there is a type of qi stagnation. People with qi stagnation constituion are vulnerable to depression, which is related to the innate nature of personality disorders. TCM considers that any stagnation is based on illness of visceral qi, for which excessive worrying combined with weakness in viscera lead to six stagnations.

Illness of visceral qi refers to depression caused by prenatal visceral qi. It is inborn with personality traits of being introverted, emotionally unstable, depressive, melancholic, vulnerable, sensitive, susceptible, paranoid and indifferent. Illness of visceral qi shares similar clinical manifestations with depression. In terms of TCM, patients with illness of visceral qi are characterized by being slim, melancholy, lack of vitality, distending sensation and pain in the chest and hypochondrium, sighing, globus sensation, loss of appetite, poor memory, light red tongue coating, wiry and thin pulse. People with qi stagnation constituion are vulnerable to depression. In cloudy and rainy days, they would feel gloomy with tightness in chest. Although depression is not a genetic disorder, it is highly related to family medical history. According to statistics, 30%–41.8% patients with depression have family history of psychiatric illness. Those who have relatives with depression are 10–30 times more vulnerable than normal people to depression. I met many patients with digestive diseases accompanied by depression and asked them whether their parents had history of psychiatric illness, depression, or anxiety disorders. They said yes. Increased noradrenaline release can make people easily get anxious, while depletion of noradrenaline can make people vulnerable to depression. Increased noradrenaline release pertains to yang syndrome, while depletion of noradrenaline pertains to yin syndrome, in terms of TCM. Clinical research found that to warm the kidney and tonify yang can help relieve depression.

In recent years, many newly published books inspired me a lot. When I treated patients with digestive diseases accompanied by depression, I used the ingredients that can soothe liver qi and unblock and warm yang, especially kidney yang, which could increase noradrenaline release. That was actually the contribution of integrated traditional Chinese and Western medicine.

(2) Psychosocial factors.

They involve life events or bad experience. In Western medicine, personality disorders are regarded as internal factors and psychosocial factors as external factors. However, TCM takes psychosocial factors as internal causes of disease.

But TCM and Western medicine do have some opinions in common. There are two concepts regarding the causes of stagnation syndrome in TCM, that is, stagnation leading to disease and disease leading to stagnation. Stagnation leading to disease is about psychosocial factors causing stagnation syndrome, involving life events and long-term unpleasant experience. That is a functional mental illness. Disease leading to stagnation was put forward by Zhang Jingyue in Ming dynasty. In clinic, many patients have cerebral strokes, heart diseases, cancers, diabetes, stomach disorders, precancerous gastrointestinal lesions, laryngeal precancerous lesions, etc. By time, patients can have fear and get depressed, so that depression and anxiety disorders may happen, which is about disease leading to stagnation.

Psychiatric disorders can be classified into two categories, in terms of Western medicine. One is functional psychiatric disorders, which are primary, and the other is secondary psychiatric disorders, which are caused by physical illness. For example, vascular dementia is dementia caused by vascular diseases such as cerebral hemorrhage and cerebral infarction. It is regarded as disease leading to stagnation in TCM and classified as a psychiatric disorder caused by physical illness in Western medicine.

The categorization in Western medicine is consistent with stagnation leading to disease and disease leading to stagnation put forward by Zhang Jingyue. It is astonishing that Zhang found the rules hundreds of years ago. In the following, I will further analyze yin and yang properties in depression and anxiety disorders. TCM holds "patience pertains to yin and restlessness pertains to yang," with static yin contradictory to dynamic yang. Depression belongs to yin syndrome, featured by silence and introversion, while anxiety disorders belong to yang syndrome, featured by hyperactivity, agitation and restlessness.

The Original Meaning of Cold Damage (*Shāng Hán Yuán Zhĭ*, 伤寒原旨) by He Rukui in Qing dynasty reads that "if yin does not fuse with yang, yang would overact, and if yang does not fuse with yin, yin would curdle." So yin and yang must interact with each other so that the harmony of yin and yang can be reached. Regarding psychiatry, there are also yin syndrome and yang syndrome. For schizophrenia, the types with mania belong to yang syndrome, while the types with silence belong to yin syndrome. Likewise, depression belongs to yin syndrome and anxiety disorders belong to yang syndrome, based on their signs and symptoms. The reason behind is that depression involves sadness, retarded thinking, and inertia. Futhermore, regarding its pathogenesis, depression pertains to wood and the liver. Based on the theory of five phases, wood, among metal, wood, water, fire and earth, corresponds to the liver, among the liver, heart, spleen, lung and kidney. Liver qi must flow smoothly. If liver qi is stagnated, it can turn into depression by time, which can be treated by soothing liver qi and activating blood. The liver stores blood so unsmooth flow of blood in the liver can block the collaterals of liver and then bring damage to liver functions. At last, cirrhosis can occur. TCM literature records that "when people are lying down, their blood flows back to the liver, and when they are walking, the blood flows through the meridians and collaterals all over the body." That is to say, when people are sleeping at night, blood is stored in the liver; when they are moving, blood goes around the body from the liver. That is a dynamic process and blood in the liver flows. So in clinical practice, TCM would soothe liver qi and activate blood to relieve liver qi stagnation and treat hepatic diseases. Liver Research Institute in Shanghai University of Traditional Chinese Medicine invented Fuzheng Huayu Jiaonang (扶正化瘀胶囊, Capsule for reinforcing the healthy qi and removing stasis) to treat cirrhosis, by soothing and nourishing the liver as well as dissolving and removing stasis.

Anxiety disorders belong to yang syndrome, with three major signs including nervousness, psychomotor agitation, and autonomic hyperactivity. Depression pertains to the liver and wood, while anxiety disorders pertain to fire. Fire is hot, with its property of flaming upward. People with flamed fire would have redness on face. Anxiety disorders pertain to fire, manifested by hyperactivity, agitation and restlessness. TCM classifies the fire into sovereign fire and ministerial fire. What is sovereign fire then? Heart pertains to fire, so heart fire is named sovereign fire. Among the five zang-organs of heart, liver, spleen, lung and kidney, the heart governs physiological functions of zang-fu organs. If yang qi is insufficient, heart blood stasis and obstruction could occur so that myocardial infarction may happen in a severe condition. So patients with myocardial infarction should be treated by warming yang, activating blood, and dissipating cold. When yang qi is sufficient, blood in vessels would flow smoothly. Why are there so many cases of myocardial infarction in winter? That is because there is less yang qi in winter. Besides, the elderly have insufficient original yang, so they usually have cold limbs. When it comes to the midnight, weak yang qi with insufficient fire qi slow down the flow of blood and cause blockage, leading to pain or even death in a severe condition. So myocardial infarction must be treated by warming yang and activating blood. Therefore, TCM uses Shexiang Baoxin Wan (麝香保心丸, Moschus Heart-Protecting Pill) to activate blood and resolve stasis, and relieve blockage with aroma.

Fire can be categorized into deficiency fire and excess fire. Liver-kidney yin deficiency can cause fire, but such fire is deficiency fire. When people catch a cold and a fever, accompanied by pneumonia with body temperature of around 40°C, that is excess fire. In Western medicine, antibiotics are used to manage inflammation, while in TCM, Chinese herbal formulas are prescribed to clear and purge excess fire. Some people have yin deficiency, dry mouth, dry stools, palm burning sensation, redness on face, and warm sensations throughout body with sweating, which are manifestations of yin deficiency with effulgent fire. Those can be treated by nourishing yin and clearing fire. It may sound abstract, but it does work in clinical practice and benefit patients, based on the principle of syndrome differentiation and treatment. Where there is warm body temperature, there is heat; where there is heat, there is fire. For deficiency fire, antibiotics do not work, but TCM can nourish yin and downbear fire to restore health.

9.4.2. Disease mechanism of stagnation syndrome

Stagnation syndrome mainly involves the liver because the liver pertains to wood. Patients with depression have liver qi stagnation. They are sleepy and lack of vitality because there are congealed phlegm clouding clear yang, and oppressed spirit qi in their bodies. There are three types of fire in anxiety disorders, including liver stagnation transforming into fire, liver-kidney yin deficiency leading to yin deficiency with effulgent fire, and non-interaction between the heart and kidney. The heart pertains to heart fire and the kidney pertains to water. Normally, water of yin and fire of yang are supposed to reach balance. When yin and yang are imbalanced, leading to non-interaction between the heart and kidney, insomnia, restlessness and agitation would occur. So, anxiety disorders involve three categories of fire, including liver fire, yin deficiency with effulgent fire, and non-interaction between the heart and kidney. Each category has corresponding treatments in clinical practice.

9.4.3 Treatment for stagnation syndrome

To treat depression, TCM focuses on soothing the liver, improving qi, resolving phlegm, unblocking yang and relieving stagnation. Xiaoyao San (逍遥散, Peripatetic Powder) can soothe liver qi. It makes people feel released by relieving liver qi stagnation. Chaihu Shugan San (柴胡疏肝散, Bupleurum Liver-Soothing Powder) and Wendan Tang (温胆汤, Gallbladder-Warming Decoction) are the alternatives. In clinical practice, I usually add Guizhi (桂枝, Ramulus Cinnamomi), Xixin (细辛, Herba Asari), and Xianlingpi (仙灵脾, Herba Epimedii) to improve therapeutic effects, unblocking yang and relieving liver stagnation.

Disease mechanism of anxiety disorders is based on fire, so to clear fire is important during treatment. Dan Zhi Xiaoyao San (丹栀逍遥散, Peripatetic Powder with Cortex Moutan and Fructus Gardneiae) and Zhi Bai Xiaoyao San (知柏逍遥散, Peripatetic Powder with Rhizoma Anemarrhenae and Cortex Phellodendri) can treat liver stagnation transforming into fire. Zhi Bai Dihuang Wan (知柏地黄丸, Six-Ingredient Rehmannia Pill with Rhizoma Anemarrhenae and Cortex Phellodendri) and Da Buyin Wan (大补阴丸, Major Yin Tonifying Pill) can treat liver-kidney yin deficiency with effulgent fire. If practitioners of Western medicine learn the basics of TCM, they can also prescribe TCM patent medicines. Ejiao Jizihuang Tang (阿胶鸡子黄汤, Ass Hide Glue and Egg Yolk Decoction) with Huanglian (黄连, Rhizoma Coptidis) can treat non-interaction between the heart and kidney, in which egg yolks have therapeutic effects on non-interaction between the heart and kidney, insomnia, restlessness and anxiety.

Besides, a medicinal cuisine Jieyu Wangyou Tang (解郁忘忧汤, Stagnation-Relieving and Grief-Forgetting Decoction) is recommended, containing Huanghuacai (黄花菜, Hemerocallis citrina Baroni) also named daylily. The formula consists of daylily, flowers with the action of soothing liver qi, including Hehuanhua (合欢花, Flos Albiziae), Meiguihua (玫瑰花, Flos Rosae Rugosae), Daidaihua (代代花, Flos Citri Aurantii Amarae), 3 grams of Lianzixin (莲子心, Plumula Nelumbinis), Baihe

(百合, Bulbus Lilii), Hongzao (红枣, Fructus Jujubae), and Gancao (甘草, Radix Glycyrrhizae), in which the lotus plumule is quite bitter. Decoct the ingredients with water into the decoction of 150ml. Take the decoction twice a day. This therapy can also be taken as an aid of treatment for patients with depression, who can take the decoction for one to two months, as a medicated diet.

Another supplementary therapy is the foot bath. Decoct Danggui (当归, Radix Angelicae Sinensis), Honghua (红花, Flos Carthami), Shichangpu (石菖蒲, Rhizoma Acori Tatarinowii), Zhenzhumu (珍珠母, Concha Margaritifera), Rougui (肉桂, Cortex Cinnamomi), Huanglian (黄连, Rhizoma Coptidis) with water. Practice foot bath in the decoction, with water temperature of 30–45°C, which can help sleep better. Both depression and anxiety disorders can lead to insomnia. About 90% of patients with depression and anxiety disorders experienced insomnia. So, the therapy of foot bath can be taken as an aid to improve sleep.

9.5 Psychotherapy for depression

TCM literature *Categorized Patterns with Clear-cut Treatments* (*Lèi Zhèng Zhì Cái*, 类证治裁) in Qing dynasty reads "failure to realize ambition, bad experience, and accumulated grievances can cause stagnation, so original causes must be found out to remove negative thinking during treatment," putting emphasis on psychotherapy. It also reads "if bad moods cannot be relieved, with stagnation leading to damage, herbal medications would not make success." That is to say simply using medicinal herbs can not bring out satisfying therapeutic effects for diseases caused by depression and anxiety. "How can we use albizia flower to remove anger, and daylily to remove worries?" That means, simply using Hehuanhua (合欢花, Flos Albiziae) and Huanghuacai (黄花菜, Hemerocallis citrina Baroni) cannot really help with illness caused by psychological factors.

For psychotherapy, there are three principles.

The first one is to listen. For patients with depression and anxiety disorders or similar symptoms, physicians should listen to their complaints with patience. In clinical practice, some patients showed sheets of paper with their symptoms to doctors, because they have expectations of doctors and hope doctocs can fully understand their conditions. Every time I met such patients, actually I felt ashamed and I had no excuse to interrupt or ignore them because complaining itself was also a process of releasing emotions. So, no matter how busy they are, physicians must listen to patients, patiently and attentively.

The second is to relieve. Although doctors may not cure all the diseases, they can correct wrong understandings patients have. Doctors can tell patients what is right and what is wrong. For example, when patients ask if atrophic gastritis will cause stomach cancer, I would explain that only 1%–3% of atrophic gastritis would turn into stomach cancer, based on medical literature home and abroad I read and my experience of treating patients with various stomach disease over decades. So I usually reassure patients with such facts. We must correct the wrong understandings patients have. For intestinal metaplasia of the stomach and stomach dysplasia, surgery is considered when test results contain more than three "+." Normally, conservative therapies are selected when there are only two "+" in test results. There are also several TCM treatments for such problems so we need to offer explanations to patients and relieve their worries.

The third is to support. Instead of "to guarantee," I think "to support" is more appropriate. Doctors would not say "I guarantee you can be cured," but should firmly tell patients that there is no evidence of worsening by far, and it can be improved gradually with proper treatments. We should help patients to build up self-esteem, confidence in treatment and hope in life, and ask them to follow doctors' advice and have faith in the future. I had a patient with atrophic gastritis, who had been told by her previous doctor that it could turn into cancer, and later at night she got insomnia. She came to me the next day, crying and shouting because she was so anxious. I talked and explained to her with patience for a few times. Then she gradually felt mentally relieved and could have good sleep. Good sleep improved depression and anxiety disorders so that her symptoms were gradually relieved. It can be seen psychotherapy actually does not work instantly but takes time and skills.

For patients with depression or anxiety disorders, there are a few things they need pay attention to.

The first is to keep occupied. Nothing to do would empty the spirit. Many patients asked me, "you are more than 70 years old, and what is your secret to keep healthy?" I said my way of health cultivation is to keep myself occupied so that I do not have time to be sick. I have things to do so I have enriched minds. I devote all my energy to clinical practice and training students so I am too busy to be sick. Nothing to do can make people feel empty and bored, which may cause depression and anxiety disorders.

The second is to interact with people and avoid loneliness. People must have hobbies so that they can entertain themselves with something when they get old. I practice calligraphy occasionally although I am usually busy. I practice not to be an expert, but for life nurturing and emotional regulation. Professor Yi Zhongtian said, "there are two motives behind reading, one for making money and another for cultivating the mind." If a job is for making money, then practicing calligraphy is for cultivating the mind. If jobs and hobbies are balanced, physical and mental health will be maintained.

The third is to follow health care professional's instructions to take medications and take routine physical examinations. Many patients had already seen counseling psychologists before they came to me. I told them not to stop the administration or reduce the dosage of Western medication arbitrarily, and asked them to return to the psychologists for regular checkups.

The last but the most important is to maintain a healthy lifestyle. Many people with depression or anxiety disorders have difficulties restoring health because they have irregular lifestyle and know little about preservation of mental health. In clinical practice, I met a patient with a history of depression for six years. He had been using antidepressants and anti-anxiety medications. Two years ago, he committed suicide, slitting his wrist. He was rescued but still had serious symptoms of depression and anxiety disorders with mild stomach disease. I prescribed him Xiaoyao San (逍遥散, Peripatetic Powder) and modified Chaihu Shugan San (柴胡疏肝散, Bupleurum Liver-Soothing Powder) with Rhizoma Anemarrhenae and Cortex Phellodendri. After one year of the administration with psychotherapy, his symptoms have been gradually improved. Now the dosage of Western medicine is reduced to half by his psychiatrist. He can sleep for 8 hours at night, with a stable emotional state and improved gastrointestinal conditions. His depression is generally under control. I prescribed him TCM medicines intermittently and his psychiatrist reduced the dosage of western medication step by step. In this way, many patients received satisfying results.

The host: Thank you, Professor Wang Qingqi, for the brilliant speech. Other than TCM, we also would like to invite other experts to share more ideas. So, today we have Professor Wang Zhen to explain depression from the perspective of Western medicine.

Wang Zhen: Professor Wang Qingqi has just talked about depression from the perspective of TCM and I am going to explain it based on Western medicine.

From the speech of Professor Wang qingqi, I see he must be a TCM master and also a good psychotherapist. He just explained his clinical practice without terms of so-called modern science. A good psychiatrist does not have to be a good psychotherapist. There are two major academic branches in psychiatry, one of pure biology and another of combining biology and psychology. Although we consider the mode of pure biomedicine should be improved, few people can make differences, especially under the circumstances of understaffed healthcare professionals in China. On Saturday, I met a professor of ethics from the United States. He asked me, "what are differences do you think between psychiatrists in China and the United States?" I said an obvious difference lies in that, for half a day, a psychiatrist in China may see more than 30 patients while a psychiatrist in the United States would see about three or four patients. Nowadays in china, it might be hard to change the overall medicine mode, but integrated TCM and western medicine can be practiced to be a great psychiatrist since TCM puts emphasis on both physical and mental health. Actually, I am quite interested in how TCM looks at emotions. What Professor Wang Qingqi just introduced to us reminds us of the fact that TCM does put emphasis on psychotherapy and psychological counselling. Personally, I believe there are effective therapies in TCM to treat psychological disorders. I did researches on anxiety disorders and tried to find theoretical support in TCM for the treatment for anxiety disorders. Biologically, there are not many differences in depression between China and the US, but culturally there are. Many comparative researches home and abroad have an interesting result that there are more physical symptoms among patients in China than in the Western countries. Although theoretically patients with depression should see psychiatrists and psychologists, more than 40% of them went to departments of TCM and internal medicine.

Among patients in the departments of digestive health, cardiology and neurology, 30%–35% fully match the diagnostic criteria of anxiety disorders and depression. But if their doctors tell them they have mental problems, they may have complaints. Besides, I am very interested in "shanghuo (get fire)" in TCM mentioned before, but I haven't found any related theoretical support. I think it might be related to anxiety. And for "fire" causing toothache in TCM, Western medicine actually cannot give a diagnosis if there is no infection. I stayed in the US for two years. It would be difficult to explain "fire" to the Americans because there is no corresponding concept in Western medicine. Probably psychology can provide an explanation so we can combine psychology with TCM. It is of great significance and much fun to do research on "shanghuo (get fire)" in TCM. I would like to advise TCM experts to do such research and find out what exactly the mechanism is behind it. It might be related to endocrine, but not inflammation caused by bacterial infection. Some of the contents I was going to talk about was already covered by Professor Wang Qingqi, so I would skip the same parts.

Now I am going to talk about depression in terms of Western medicine. At the very beginning, depression was literally translated into "忧郁症 (melancholy)" in Chinese instead of "抑郁症 (depression)" because melancholy in Chinese had been frequently used in daily life. It was modified into "抑郁症" later, which is more appropriate in my opnion. Among the characters of "抑郁症," "抑" means suppression and "郁" means melancholy. So there is not only melancholy but also suppression in depression. Melancholy refers to a state, while suppression refers to a process. If all the activities of people are suppressed, they will have no interest in anything, and even their desire of human instincts would be gone. So, depression consists of suppression and melancholy.

"郁" in Chinese includes two meanings, depression and vitality. Depression is about suppression of all the things with vitality. At the beginning, translators did not demonstrate that, but now we can see it is more appropriate to understand in this way.

Then, I will explain depression with four parts from the perspective of Western medicine.

9.6 Definition of depression

What is depression? I will give you a few typical examples.

The first one is about Princess Diana. She had at least four depressive episodes. She once wrote, "you are not wearing my shoes so you never know how my feet are feeling." The other two examples I am going to talk about later are similar to this. Diana demonstrated her goodness in front of people but death turned out to be the best way to free herself. So, if depression is not treated, negative emotions would get worse and ultimatly patients would resort to suicide.

When Professor Wang Qingqi talked about the differences between depression and anxiety disorders, I was reminded of a conversation between me and my patients. Some patients asked me "doctor, I think I have depression, why do you diagnose me anxiety disorders?" Other patients asked me "I think I have anxiety, why do you diagnose me depression?" To put it simply, I explained to them that depression involves desire for death while anxiety disorders involve fear of death. However, when anxiety goes too far, sufferings may still push patients to commit suicide. But to them, death is only a solution but not what they pursue. So, patients with anxiety disorders may say "I cannot tolerate sufferings any more so I chose death, but I won't do so if I am free of sufferings." For patients with depression, they would say "I just wanna die because I have no other way to go."

Many people have psychological disorders because of their childhood trauma or their families. So both genes and environments can make differences. Without environments, genes alone usually won't lead to the occurrence of psychological disorders.

Another case is about Rowan Atkinson. He is a well-known comedian. Atkinson had many works making people laughing, but actually he was deeply troubled by depression. Battling depression, he still always appeared pleasing in front of people. He presented pleasure to audience, but he actually was not truly happy. So, depression with such conditions in life is also called smiling depression.

According to Professor Wang Qingqi, depression is a global health threat, soon going to top the leading causes of death among diseases. Depression is estimated to be the second leading contributor to the global burden of disease by the year of 2020, and the single largest contributor by 2030.

Many people heard of depression and many people in Shanghai know about the disease, but there are still discrimination against depression and misunderstandings about the disease. Some people may say "I am strong minded so depression will never happen to me." A tough guy with a strong mind and healthy genes may move on from a negative experience, but once the impacts go beyond what he can bear, he would fall apart like smashed glass. Actually, it is more difficult to treat this type of patients. When people look strong, they may actually hide pressure, sufferings and traumas.

9.7 Signs of depression

Depression involves not only emotions, but also physical and cognitive symptoms. At the beginning, we did not pay much attention to cognitive disorders, especially in the limited sense, but Chinese people do care more about physical manifestations. If people have negative emotions, they may not speak out, but it is easier for them to express if they have physical discomforts. For example, people would say "I have to leave because of stomachache." Children would also say "I have diarrhea" when they do not want to go for a test, and would say "I have headache" when they are reluctant to go to school. I have a colleague whose son applied not to go to school with the reason of headache but actually he had emotional problems. He had negative experience at school, so he felt anxious with headache at school. So, the reason he reported to school was a half-truth.

It is not humiliating to have physical symptoms of depression, which even could happen to kids in kindergarten and primary school, including appetite changes, sleep disorders, slow movements, and decreased vitality. Chinese cultures do not encourage people to express emotions. Many of you on site today are younger than me. The overall environment is better for Gen Z and millennials. Although the cultural environment may not encourage us to express emotions, I personally encourage you to do so. Compared to English, Chinese has less words to describe emotions since we expressed less. Then, what can we do? Patients with depression in China have various physical symptoms. A lot of factors can cause depression, including abstract factors such as delusions, failures and ungratified wishes.

In theory of needs, people have esteem needs. Depression could happen if the basic needs are not met. Broken object relations could cause feelings of guilt because people with such feelings would want to hurt, punish and destroy involved objects.

For example, although some people had quarrels with their parents, they actually did not hope to. So, they would feel guilty, leading to depressed moods. It is worth noting that some patients do have depressed moods, but they do not have to be diagnosed as depression.

About depressed moods and the disease of depression, I will explain from three aspects.

The first is about depressed moods. Everyone can experience depressed moods, lasting a few days or weeks but no longer than two weeks. Normally, depressed moods last no more than 3 days. So, three days after bad experiences, basically emotional balance should start to be restored. But it has to be taken seriously if negative moods are not relieved at all after three days.

The second is about signs of depression. Compared to depressive disorders, signs of depression cover a wider range of contents. People with signs of depression do not have to be diagnosed with depression but they do have depressed moods lasting longer than normal.

The third is about depressive disorders. People with depressive disorders meet diagnostic criteria in terms of time span, severity, etc. Besides, I actually have a question about bipolar disorder. Bipolar disorder includes episodes of depression. That is what I would like to discuss with Professor Wang Qingqi after listening to his speech. He said depression belongs to yin syndrome. Then what type of syndrome does bipolar disorder involving depression belong to?

Let's look at the symptoms of depression. Actually most symptoms of depression are covered by the above three aspects. To be more specific, the symptoms include insomnia, low self-confidence, and low self-esteem. Physical symptoms include fatigue. The most serious manifestations include negative ways of thinking, committing suicide, retarded thinking, memory loss. Many people with memory loss went to the department of neurology, complaining of poor memory. The core symptom of depression is low mood.

Other illnesses may also involve depression, such as headache, chest tightness, heart palpitations, and gastrointestinal disorders. I had many patients with gastrointestinal disorders, as well as muscle soreness. Those symptoms are most commonly seen in the middle-aged and elderly. The physical symptoms involve many systems including nervous system, respiratory system, digestive system, and urinary system.

Some people say, "You eat and sleep regularly, and how can you have depression?" A small number of patients with depression have increased appetite, long sleeping, and even weight gain. So depression cannot be ruled out even with those three manifestations. Common signs and symptoms of depression are decreased appetite, decreased sleep, and weight loss, but increased appetite can also happen.

Some people are rejection-sensitive and they may view rejection as horrible. For example, if a leave request is refused by the leader, they would feel depressive because they wonder "why can others ask for leave, but I cannot?" It is related with cognitive modes.

People with major depressive disorder would not get happy even when they encounter something exciting. Patients with mild to moderate depression are sensitive to negative events, but they still can sense happiness to some extent. So even with pleasure, depression still cannot be excluded completely.

Some cases are rarely seen in daily life but can be found in a hospital for psychiatry, such as depression with psychiatric disorders. Such patients are very paranoid, and they would think "this person is trying to harm me" if they are told something they do not like. This psychotic depression is a subtype of major depression that occurs when a severe depressive illness includes some form of psychosis. Some patients have mixed episodes. For example, a few patients with depression might have high energy for a short period of time.

The above is a general introduction to depression. Here I am not going further into bipolar disorder. Besides, there is mixed anxiety-depressive disorder, characterized by symptoms of both depression and anxiety.

Anxiety disorders involve more than temporary worry or fear, but also panic attacks, social phobia, natural environment phobias, etc. According to the latest statistics in China, prevalence of anxiety disorders is 4.63%, while prevalence of depression is 4.0%, showing that there are more cases of anxiety disorders than cases of depression. In the state of Qi there lived a man who, filled with apprehensions of the imminent fall of the sky and the consequent destruction of his hearth and home, was so vexed that he could neither eat nor sleep. The short story has been frequently used to illustrate anxiety and later to demonstrate generalized anxiety disorder. Generalized anxiety disorder symptoms include persistent worrying, instead of chest tightness or panic attacks, lasting more than six months. The man in the state of Qi could be diagnosed with generalized anxiety disorder if he had persistent worrying. He could be diagnosed with panic attacks if he had serious symptoms but with a short period of worrying. If he kept thinking about how to prevent the fall of the sky, that might be obsessive-compulsive disorder. Obsessive-compulsive disorder (OCD) is a common anxiety disorder. When I became a physician at the beginning, I thought depression could be completely separated from anxiety disorders. With more clinical practice, I have found depression and anxiety disorders cannot be completely separated, which usually occur together.

Besides, it is more difficult to treat mixed anxiety-depressive disorder than to treat single anxiety or single depression. There is a higher risk of committing suicide for anxiety-depressive disorder. Although patients with depression have suicidal tendencies, actions can be delayed because they have weaker motives when their depression is too severe. However, patients with anxiety-depressive disorder would have more tendencies to commit suicide because of anxiety, so there is a higher risk of committing suicide.

9.8 Treatment for depression

Lastly, how do we treat depression? Women are vulnerable to depression. In China, there are more female than male patients with depression asking for treatment. That does not mean men are mentally stronger because they tend to choose tolerance. Once men mentally get sick, the conditions are usually very serious. Women with physiological and psychological sufferrings are more vulnerable to depression. Stress is also a contributor to depression. Why do people nowadays especially in big cities easily get sick? One main reason is extreme stress. There are various sources of stress. There are stress at work, stress of promotion, homework stress, stress from parents and teachers. So, the prevalence of depression among students is increasing.

More and more people in China have childhood trauma. Childhood trauma includes not only physical abuse but also emotional neglect. For example, there are leftover children, who are left in their hometowns in the countryside, with parents going out to earn money. Although there are not many leftover children in Shanghai, children raised by grandparents or nannies can also have childhood trauma. They are more vulnerable to depression and anxiety disorders when they grow up. Another situation is depression caused by disease, corresponding to disease leading to stagnation in TCM.

Then when should we be careful? Normally everyone can experience emotional change. No matter it is sadness or happiness, they generally would disappear in three days. Three is only an estimated but not absolute number. If sadness is not relieved for even a little bit in three days, that is to say, if stimuli disappear but you still feel stuck in negative emotions, you would better ask for help from professionals. For instance, you keep feeling stuck after a breakup, or you have severe depressed moods for a few months after big property losses. Generally, if handled properly in three days, depressed moods would be eliminated gradually to some extent. If depressed moods last longer than two weeks and even get worse, it is better to go to a professional, according to clinical criteria.

Statistics two years ago showed 800 thousand people died of depression leading to suicide every year. This number might be a little smaller than the factual one because people who died of car accidents include some who died of depression leading to suicide. Some people with depression ran into the road and were killed by car accidents, which were finally recorded as car accident deaths. In some cases of disease leading to depression, families of patients did not want others know they committed suicide and would declare that they died of heart attacks, which was finally recorded as death from disease.

When you face the following situations, you need to be very careful because they imply risks of committing suicide. That is talking about committing suicide. Most people would tell others about their suicidal thoughts before they are to do so. I had a patient aged 18 or 19 years old, who was rescued after committing suicide. Before he committed suicide, he had asked what he could do to die peacefully. His mom replied to him a kid should not speak of death. The mom did not care about that, and the patient committed suicide the second day in a way found online. Some people would even take sleeping pills to kill themselves. So, we are very cautious about prescribing sleeping pills unless patients have the history of confirmed disease. Another situation is to pay too much attention to life and death with desperation. Besides, what is easily ignored is sudden silence. If someone has been always complaining "I am so upset and I can't handle" but suddenly becomes silent, it must be taken seriously to find out the reasons behind.

An elderly patient was hospitalized for treatment. At the beginning, he kept complaining everyday that "I am dying...I am dying..." His symptoms were improved gradually after taking medicines. One day he suddenly got fine emotionally, and stopped complaining about dying or his kids. From his eyes and facial expressions, we could see that he was not so good as he told us. Then, I told his nurses that they needed to pay more attention to him because he might not be so good as he showed to us. At that noon, he said he wanted to go back home. I refused because it took too many risks. But his families came and said they would look after him. To respect the patient and his families, I agreed to let him go back. But that was actually the calm before the storm. After going back home, the patient took a new haircut, put on decent clothing and then committed suicide.

Then, is it possible to completely cure depression? Personally, I don't think a disease can be completely cured because no one can be sure that there will no recurrence of the disease. There are ways to treat depression, but we cannot completely cure it. Why does depression impress people with difficulties in treating depression socially and clinically? Because many people think it can reoccur frequently. In fact, many patients did not follow doctor's advice to receive treatment or prevent relapse. If a medication works well, we usually advise patients to take it for 1–2 years, at least 1 year. And to stop taking medications at a proper time is quite important. For example, if patients start administration at a certain season and the symptoms are relieved for one year, with the overall situation improved, it is not advised to stop administration because biological characteristics must be taken into consideration. To stop administration and treatment in a proper season and at a right time is very important. Generally speaking, poor obedience of patients towards taking suggested medicines is one main reason behind the relapse of depression. Nowadays, when physicians get to know the situations of patients, they usually remind patients not to stop administration arbitually and advise them to follow doctor's advice strictly.

For treatment, I mainly explained from the perspective of biology with focus on medications. But actually in clinical practice, psychological treatment is significant. The differences between doctors does not only lie in medications. Different physicians prescribe the same drugs but they would have different effects because they practice psychotherapy in different ways.

In many cases, communicating with patients in a sincere way with reliable information can restore their confidence. I had a patient from other provinces. He had seen doctors locally for no more than 3 weeks. When he came to me, his symptoms were actually improved. He had asked the local doctor if he could be cured. The doctor replied that it was hard to say and the relapse rate was high. He came to me and asked if he could be cured. I was writing a case history. Then, I looked up at him and said sure. I did not mean to lie to him. I looked into his eyes with sincerity and told him he could be treated. He refused to take the drug prescribed by the previous doctor, so I prescribed a new one, but actually both have similar mechanism. Two weeks later, he told me my prescription was better. I knew it was actually my words that cheered him up.

So, we can see that confidence and trust are very important. When we have confidence, body functions may be activated to fight against depression. Medications alone would not make satisfying effects. And it is almost impossible to cure anxiety disorders caused by psychological factors simply through medications. There are many treatments based on biology, including physical therapy, magnetic field therapy, and electroconvulsive therapy. There are also many researches on developing new drugs. We are looking forward to more remedies for depression in the future.

LECTURE 10

Add Firewood to Flames

TCM Culture and Health Preservation

LECTURER: WANG QINGQI

Introduction to the speaker:

Wang Qingqi is a tenured professor in Shanghai University of Traditional Chinese Medicine, with the title of Shanghai Famous TCM Doctor. Entitled to special government allowances from the State Council in China, he is an academic experience inheritance instructor of national outstanding TCM experts, who has trained 40 students including PhD students, post-doctoral fellows and academic inheritors. He is also an editor-in-chief of TCM for *Chinese Dictionary of Etymology* (*Ci Hai*, 辞海). Prof. Wang has been engaged in the practice of TCM internal medicine (involving digestive diseases and psychosomatic disorders) and in teaching *The Inner Canon of the Yellow Emperor* (*Huáng Dì Nèi Jīng*, 黄帝内经) for over 50 years. He has been the editor-in-chief and the associate editor-in-chief for more than 50 academic books. He won the first prize of Shanghai TCM Science and Technology Awards and the second prize of China Association of Chinese Medicine Science and Technology Award. Besides, he is the host of TCM Psychology Master Studio funded by Shanghai Municipal Education Commission.

Traditional Chinese medicine (TCM), born in China, perfectly combines traditional Chinese culture with natural science. Cultures of the Chinese nation are extensive and profound, which have been well preserved, delicately integrating culture into natural science. Many countries, including ancient Greece, Arabia, and India, have their own traditional medicine. However, some of the traditional medicine in those countries has been taken as folk medicine after the 21st century, with modern medicine being the mainstream, and some only have insignificant formulas and skills preserved. Most of them have not been taken as important medical resources in the countries. TCM is considered as important as western medicine and is significant in disease prevention and treatment in China. In recent decades, with the implementation of China's "Going Out" strategy, TCM has spread to more than 140 countries and regions around the world.

10.1 The definition of culture

Traditional Chinese medicine combines culture and medicine perfectly. Then, what is culture?

Economy and culture are two basic forms of human activities, which together contributes to continuous progress and development of human society. The remarkable mark that distinguishes human beings from animals is that animals only have material needs but not spiritual needs; apart from material needs, human beings also have spirits, morals, ideals, wisdom and so on, which refers to culture. Therefore, culture is a significant mark to distinguish animals from humans.

There are more than 400 definitions of culture in the world. Four representative definitions are listed here. Among them, what I firmly believe is a sentence in *The Scriptures of Change* (*Yì Jing*, 易经) that "look at humanity, and educate the world." It means to educate people through observing humanistic phenomena. In terms of function, culture is to cultivate and educate people with humanistic spirit. According to Hu Shi, culture refers to lifestyle, which explains culture based on the formation of culture. The culture of Chinese nation is the culture of Chinese lifestyle. In terms of connotation, culture is not an empty or abstract, which can substantially shape human personality. For example, a cultivated person depends not on university education background but on personality and behavior.

According to Xi Jinping, general secretary of the Communist Party of China Central Committee, "Chinese culture bears the ultimate spirit the Chinese nation pursues." It involves the function of culture.

10.2 Culture of Traditional Chinese medicine

Traditional Chinese medicine (TCM) is a part of Chinese culture, so what is TCM culture? There are different opinions on the definition of TCM culture in academic circles. But from my point of view, TCM refers to how Chinese people live and survive. In ancient times, there was no Western medicine in China. How did Chinese people survive and reproduce? They had to fight against nature and disease. Chinese people have been struggling against disease for thousands of years, which brings TCM. Traditional Chinese medicine is concerned with the experience of how Chinese people lived and survived, which actually involves culture. Therefore, TCM culture embodies Chinese lifestyle. In the past, some people opposed traditional Chinese medicine. But Yu Qiuyu once said, "if there was no traditional Chinese medicine, how did Chinese people survive?" Western medicine was introduced into China not before 200 years ago, so before then Chinese people mainly depended on traditional Chinese medicine to treat disease. In my view, TCM culture, based on traditional Chinese culture, interprets how TCM looks at health, disease, life and death. What are the values of traditional Chinese medicine? In my opinion, the values of TCM are about how TCM explains health, disease, life and death based on traditional Chinese culture. Medicine concerns human. Humans live in nature and society at the same time. In addition, people have minds. Therefore, medicine involves nature, society and psychology. *The Inner Canon of the Yellow Emperor* (*Huáng Dì Nèi Jīng*, 黄帝内经) discusses the law of human life as well as disease prevention and treatment under the circumstances of nature and society, which is what TCM is about. My teacher, TCM master, Qiu Peiran, said that "medicine is about human." Professor Wand Weiping in Fudan University holds the same view as my teacher, who thinks medicine is the study of human beings and human life, constituting TCM culture.

TCM culture and traditional Chinese culture are so profound. Then, how can we understand TCM culture?

According to Professor Zhang Dainian in the Department of philosophy in Peking University, there are two major unique contributions TCM culture makes to human beings. One is the concept of "unity of nature and human." Qian Mu also held the same view. He believed that the greatest contribution TCM culture made to the world was the concept of "unity of nature and human." There is a viewing platform in the Chinese University of Hong Kong, right next to Victoria Harbour. The view of "unity of nature and human" by Qian Mu is engraved on the wall of the viewing platform. Another is the theory of interpersonal harmony in TCM which puts emphasis on harmony. These two contributions are actually the most important core concepts of TCM and recorded in *The Inner Canon of the Yellow Emperor* (*Huáng*

Dì Nèi Jīng, 黄帝内经), laying the foundation for theories and clinical practice of TCM.

10.3 The thought of "harmony"

The thought of "harmony" was created not by TCM, but by traditional Chinese culture, which is a representative view of Confucianism. Confucianists took impartiality and moderation as the highest moral standard and the basic principle of behavior, and first put forward the idea of "harmony as priority." Harmony has broad connotations. There are two ideas the harmony refers to.

1) "Harmony generates lives." According to Discourses of The States (Guó Yǔ, 国语), "harmony of difference generates lives, but being identical does not." That is to say, two things with different natures coexisting harmoniously can produce new things. There is a classic saying in *The Inner Canon of the Yellow Emperor* (*Huáng Dì Nèi Jīng*, 黄帝内经) that "yin and yang being harmonious generate children." Men pertain to yang and women pertain to yin. The combination of yang essence and yin essence is based on "harmony," that is, getting along harmoniously. A man and a woman get along well, so they can have affections. Then they would have children. This is about "harmony generates lives." The combination of two identical things only increases quantity, which does not produce new things. This idea is important in *The Inner Canon of the Yellow Emperor* (*Huáng Dì Nèi Jīng*, 黄帝内经) and traditional Chinese medicine. According to *The Inner Canon of the Yellow Emperor* (*Huáng Dì Nèi Jīng*, 黄帝内经), human life results from the combination of yang Qi and yin Qi, namely the combination of father essence and mother blood. "Spirit happens when two essence interact," which means that yin essence and yang essence are combined to produce new life.

2) "There is harmony in diversity." "Harmony" embodies the unity of diverse things with different characteristics. Chinese people regard nature as a unity. Humans are only one kind of things in the world. So, it is important that humans and nature keep harmonious. There are 56 ethnic groups in the Chinese nation, with 56 types of lifestyle and 56 forms of culture. They are summed up as the Chinese national culture. Each nation can maintain its own cultural characteristics, as a part of Chinese culture. A TCM prescription can contain more than ten ingredients, each of which has its own characteristics. In accordance with the hierarchy involving sovereign, minister, assistant and courier, ingredients can work harmoniously to produce new therapeutic effects for treatment. There are many

kinds of musical instruments from both the East and the West in a concert. They are combined harmoniously according to rhythm to produce wonderful music. When cooking, chefs combine all kinds of ingredients with different flavors in a certain proportion. Those are all about "harmony in diversity," which contains the great wisdom of reason. On the one hand, harmony must be maintained, and on the other hand, different things can have their own characteristics. This is an important concept that makes China such a big country unified. So, I think this idea is very great.

Then, what is "harmony" in TCM? If you get to know traditional Chinese medicine from the basis, you can immediately understand its core ideas, otherwise it always sounds mysterious about TCM. To learn TCM culture can help better understand that TCM is not a pseudo-science but a subject of philosophical knowledge revealing the thinking mode of Oriental people. Then, how does TCM interpret physiology, pathology, disease prevention and treatment with the thought of "harmony"?

(1) THE DEFINITION OF HEALTH IN THE THOUGHT OF "HARMONY"

Let's take a look at how traditional Chinese medicine understands health. A Western medicine practitioner once asked me, "we have a global criterion for health in Western medicine, and do you have a criterion for health in traditional Chinese medicine?" I said yes and explained with the viewpoints in *The Inner Canon of the Yellow Emperor* (*Huáng Dì Nèi Jīng*, 黄帝内经) and *The Divine Pivot* (*Líng Shū*, 灵枢) · The Viscera as The Foundation of Human Beings, that the essence of health is "harmony," which includes three aspects. The first one is "harmony of Qi and blood." Traditional Chinese medicine attaches importance to Qi and blood, which are basic materials to constitute and maintain human life. The second one is "harmony between mind and body," namely the harmony of physiology and psychology. The third is "harmony between human and nature." In short, health refers to a harmonious state between human and nature, psychology and physiology, Qi and blood, in TCM. There are also three criteria for health in Western medicine. The first one is physically not being sick. The second is normal mental state. The third is a sound state with proper social adaptation. Those are actually similar to the criteria for health in TCM. But the "harmony" contains more profound connotations. What does the sound state in Western medicine mean? There is no perfectly sound person, so actually there is no exact definition of sound person. The concept of "harmony" in TCM is with more sense of philosophy than the description of the sound state.

(2) THE THOUGHT OF "HARMONY" AND DISEASE

Pathogenic factors can break the harmony between human and nature, psychology and physiology, Qi and blood, and then cause various symptoms and signs of diease physically and mentally. From the perspective of Western medicine, what causes disease? It includes biological factors such as viruses and bacteria, as well as physical and chemical factors. Besides, mental factors also make differences. Nowadays, mental stress is an important cause of disease. There are many functional disorders and organic diseases caused by psychological factors, accounting for 1/3 – 2/3 of all discases. For example, cardiovascular diseases, cerebrovascular diseases, malignant tumors and diabetes are all related to psychological factors. External and internal pathogenic factors invade human body, which destroys the harmonious state between human and nature, psychology and physiology, Qi and blood, thus showing various symptoms, from the perspective of TCM. TCM puts emphasis on "syndrome differentiation and treatment." Specifically, there are two key points of "syndrome differentiation and treatment." One is to identify causes of disease based on clinical manifestations. The other is to determine body constitution. Everyone has a unique body constitution, and different constitutions have different responses to pathogenic factors. From the perspective of Western medicine, disease refers to the response of body to pathogenic factors. From the perspective of TCM, pathogenic factors break harmony in three aspects, leading to a variety of physical symptoms or signs, namely, disease.

(3) THE THOUGHT OF "HARMONY" AND TREATMENT

The process of "syndrome differentiation and treatment" is to identify the causes of disease and body constitution, to make a diagnosis, and then to determine treatment principles. For example, aversion to cold, frequent urination at night in winter, soreness around the waistline and legs, dizziness, tinnitus, vertigo are signs of kidney deficiency in TCM. So the treatment is to tonify the kidney. The treatment principle is to remove disharmony and restore health, based on "syndrome differentiation." When I was learning from Professor Qiu peiran, he once asked me, "What are the characteristics of TCM in your opinion based on your experience of practicing TCM for almost 50 years?" I thought for a moment and said, "As people often say, the characteristic of TCM is to regulate." And what does TCM regulate? It regulates those in disharmony. Professor Deng Tietao, a TCM master, once explained with the example that a good table is very stable on the floor. Different lengths of leg can make the table instable. "Syndrome differentiation and treatment" in TCM is to find out which leg breaks harmony and to restore balance. If one leg is short, we can put a piece of wood under that leg to restore balance. Regulation aims to bring the health state close to normal, so as to achieve harmony, which can improve the quality of life for patients. There are three major treatments for cancers in Western medicine, surgery, radiotherapy and chemotherapy. Treatments of Western medicine mainly aim at local lesions. However, a cancer is taken as a local disease in TCM. For example, liver cancer is located in the liver, but such a local disease is the manifestation of systemic imbalance. Therefore, different from Western medicine, TCM regulates the overall body. There is a "seed and soil" theory of cancers in the United States, with seed referring to cancer cells, and soil referring to human body. Cancer cells fall into the soil of liver to grow, develop, reproduce, and finally form a tumor, liver cancer coming into being. Western medicine believes that the tumor is a local lesion, so treatment is to cut it off, and then targeted therapy is used to prevent metastasis and relapse. TCM believes that "where the evil gathers, healthy Qi must be deficient." The reason why people get sick is because the deficiency of healthy Qi gives pathogens chances to cause disease. First of all, the overall condition of a patient is deficient, with cancer at a local area with excess syndrome. In TCM, tumors imply blood stasis, cancer-causing toxin, phlegm dampness and other toxins gathering in the liver. Therefore, TCM treatment is to reinforce healthy qi and eliminate pathogenic factors. Academician Tang Zhaoyou of Zhongshan Hospital wrote a book *Simultaneous Elimination and Rebuilding* (*Xiāo Miè Yǔ Gǎi Zào Bìng Jǔ*, 消灭与改造并举), sharing great insights. Elimination is to remove liver cancer cells with surgery, and to remove local lesions with targeted therapy. Rebuilding is to improve the overall immunity to prevent relapse and metastasis. The main cause of death in patients with liver cancer is liver failure caused by cancer recurrence and metastasis, and failure of involved organs. In TCM, "reinforcing healthy qi and eliminating pathogenic factors" is to remove tumors by surgery, and then regulate the body through reinforcing healthy qi and improving disease resistance to prevent recurrence and metastasis. Academician Tang Zhaoyou also thinks it is reasonable to reinforce healthy qi and eliminate pathogenic factors. The so-called rebuilding is about the overall regulation, for which TCM has great potential. On the one hand, TCM can assist radiotherapy, chemotherapy and surgery, increasing therapeutic effects and reducing side effects. On the other hand, it can prevent cancer metastasis through reinforcing healthy qi. This is not contradictory to the "seed and soil" theory. Therefore, treatments in TCM and Western medicine share similarities when it comes to certain aspects, because both TCM and Western medicine aim to restore health after all, achieveing the same goal through different ways though. In short, TCM treatments originated from traditional Chinese culture.

(4) THE THOUGHT OF "HARMONY" AND HEALTH PRESERVATION

Health preservation is to prevent disease before getting sick. In TCM, the key to health preservation is to maintain the harmony between human and nature, the harmony between mind and body, and the harmony between Qi and blood, which are fundamental purposes of health preservation. It is not only about medicine, but also cultural wisdom. In short, culture and medicine are integrated in traditional Chinese medicine. Many ideas in *The Inner Canon of the Yellow Emperor* (*Huáng Dì Nèi Jīng*, 黄帝内经) and many TCM concepts are philosophical. Mr. Feng Youlan is a famous professor in the department of philosophy of Peking University. In his book, *New Edition of History of Chinese philosophy* (*Zhōng Guó Zhé Xué Shǐ Xīn Biān*, 中国哲学史新编), there is a part about *The Inner Canon of the Yellow Emperor* (*Huáng Dì Nèi Jīng*, 黄帝内经). Ren Jiyu, director of Institute for World Religions of Chinese Academy of Social Sciences, director of National Library of China, and philosopher, wrote a book *History of Chinese philosophy* (*Zhōng Guó Zhé Xué Shǐ*, 中国哲学史), in which there is a chapter on *The Inner Canon of the Yellow Emperor* (*Huáng Dì Nèi Jīng*, 黄帝内经). After reading those books, I found that some philosophers have studied Chinese medicine more deeply than doctors. Therefore, to truly understand TCM, one must learn TCM culture from the very beginning, because medicine and culture are inseparable in TCM.

The wisdom of Chinese philosophy is embodied in the word "harmony." It not only stands for the basic spirit and characteristics of the Chinese nation, but also the highest value standard of Chinese philosophy and Chinese culture. Chinese government also attaches great importance to traditional culture. To revitalize China and traditional Chinese medicine, we must firstly revitalize Chinese culture. To maintain a harmonious society, to achieve peace worldwide, and to reach reconcilation between the mainland China and Taiwan must follow "harmony" in the traditional culture. Dong Zhongshu is a famous philosopher in the Western Han dynasty. His wrote *Supplement to Spring and Autumn Annals* (*Chūn Qiū Fán Lù*, 春秋繁露) · Yin and Yang of Heaven and Earth, reading "the beauty of heaven and earth is no more than harmony." That means harmony generates beauty. Dishamony causes natural disasters, which destroys the beauty. *Tao Te Ching* (*Dào Dé Jīng*, 道德经) reads, "the sage makes efforts but do not dispute; the heaven does not fight but prevail; and no war overcomes harmony." Chinese philosophers think, dispute is the manifestation of contradiction, and "harmony" is the essence of contradiction. The wisdom and future of human beings lie in mastering the rules as well as understanding how to deal with yin and yang, reconcile contradictions, and promote the spirit of harmony between heaven and earth. General secretary Xi Jinping put emphasis on the thought of "harmony" in his speech that the world needs peace, but not wars. Wars will destroy the earth, and ultimately destroy human beings. According to Russell, a Western philosopher, "modern world urgently needs supreme ethical qualities of China, among which harmony is the priority that can bring more joy and peace to the earth."

After the reform and opening up, the Communist Party of China Central Committee proposed to make Chinese culture go abroad. There are a lot of treasures in traditional Chinese culture. We need to share them with other countries. There are many Confucius Institutes around the world and what they spread is traditional Chinese culture.

10.4 "Unity of nature and human"

You probably heard of "unity of nature and human," but may not understand it. Let's look at this idea from the perspective of medicine. Chinese people have been thinking about the following questions for thousands of years. How did the heaven come into being? How did human life come into being? What is the relationship between heaven and humans? These questions have been there for more than 5000 years. Therefore, traditional Chinese culture and Chinese philosophy are actually about heaven and humans. Traditional Chinese culture can be regarded as the study of heaven and humans, based on the opinions of many philosophers. I will explain how TCM embodies this concept.

(1) TCM LITERATURE ON "UNITY OF NATURE AND HUMAN"

How does *The Inner Canon of the Yellow Emperor* (*Huáng Dì Nèi Jīng*, 黄帝内经) explain the relationship between the heaven and human beings? There is a very incisive saying in the book that "the human body is closely related to the heaven and the earth and corresponds to the sun and the moon." That is to say, humans and nature are a unified whole, and people is only a part of the universe. Wang Chong, a scientist in the Eastern Han dynasty, said "weather changes in the heaven, and creatures follow on the earth." Shanghai has four seasons, spring, summer, autumn and winter. Once the weather gets cold in winter, there are many patients with cerebral infarction, myocardial infarction, tracheitis, asthma, high fever, diarrhea and stomachache in the emergency room. Why? Because "weather changes in the heaven, and creatures follow on the earth," that is to say, humans and nature are related. Failure to stay harmonious with nature makes people sick. If weather suddenly turns cold, people who are in good health can manage by taking on more pieces of cloth. However, those who are not in good health may have fever, asthma etc., even though they take on more clothes because they can't adapt to natural environments properly.

As mentioned before, if the nature and human beings are not in harmony, people cannot adapt to natural environments, causing diseases. Once, I traveled with a team to Zhongdian in Yunnan province. After we arrived there, some people vomited on the first day. Some people had headaches the next day. And on the third day, some people had fevers and couldn't eat. Those were altitude sickness. People in good health have no discomfort, eating and sleeping well. One third of the elderly in the team just slept in the hotel, unable to continue traveling, implying disharmony between humans and nature.

There is an incisive saying in *Old Book of The Tang (Jiù Táng Shū, 旧唐书)* · *Sun Si Miao* that "those who are good at explaining the heaven must understand humans well." That is to say, people who know nature well always relate it to people. "Those who are good at explaining humans also take the heaven into consideration." Both psychology and medicine are subjects of human beings. Why should we study humans based on heaven? Because human beings are actually a part of the nature, who live in natural environments. Psychology and physiology are related to not only social factors but also natural factors. If weather is fine, being sunny, moods can be pleasant. If the haze is heavy with extremely low air pressure, people may feel oppression in the chest and palpitations. Some people even have to pant, leading to gloomy and depressed moods. This is about "weather changes in the heaven, and creatures follow on the earth." Therefore, Sun Simiao was quite right. When we study human beings, what exactly do we study? It is actually nothing more than psychology and physiology. To study human beings must involve nature because human beings live in nature, not in a vacuum. Traditional Chinese medicine (TCM) is a science which takes "unity of nature and human" as its core idea to explore the law of human life.

(2) How does TCM demonstrate "unity of nature and human"?

Medicine is an applied science and a practical subject, for disease prevention and treatment. Causes of disease are related to the change of climate. No matter it is SARS or Ebola, they are both related to nature. The occurrence, development and reproduction of viruses result from the adaptability to natural environments. Therefore, to study the anti-virus and anti-bacterial treatments must involve the relationship between virus and nature, and the relationship between human body and nature. The mechanism of disease occurrence ultimately depends on whether people can adapt to natural environments, with pathogenic factors in natural environments leading to dysfunction of Qi and blood in zang-fu organs and then causing various diseases. For treatment of diseases, TCM attaches great importance to treatment based on individuals, geography, climates. Among them, treatment based on climates and geography are related to nature because climate change directly affects physiology and psychology. For example, why are people vulnerable to virus infections in cold environments? Because in a cold environment, immunity is weakened. Some researchers did an experiment. Two chickens were injected with mycobacterium tuberculosis at the same time. One chicken was raised in the natural environment, and the other was raised in a cold environment. As the result, the chicken raised in the natural environment did not get tuberculosis, but the chicken raised in the cold environment got pulmonary tuberculosis. In the cold environment, chicken immunity was weakened and mycobacterium tuberculosis were active. That is why the chicken got tuberculosis. Natural environments are closely related to health. *Basic Questions* (*Sù Wèn*, 素问) · *Discourse on how the Generative Qi Communicates with Heaven* records that vitality is yang Qi, which is closely related to nature. "Weather changes in the heaven, and creatures follow on the earth." In addition to common diseases and frequently occurring diseases, seasonal diseases are related to climate change. Women's menstruation is also closely related to the movement of celestial bodies, moon phases, as well as rise and fall of tides. Some people did research on the relationship between menstruation and moon phases, as well as rise and fall of tides recorded in *The Inner Canon of the Yellow Emperor* (*Huáng Dì Nèi Jīng*, 黄帝内经), which demonstrate "unity of nature and human" in physiology. Therefore, it is necessary to treat patients based on geography and climates.

(3) "Unity of nature and human" and health preservation

The same is true of health preservation. Different methods should be adopted in different seasons. According to *The Inner Canon of the Yellow Emperor* (*Huáng Dì Nèi Jīng*, 黄帝内经) · *Comprehensive Discourse on Regulating the Spirit in Accordance with the Qi of the Four Seasons*, different healthcare methods should be taken in four seasons of spring, summer, autumn and winter. For example, for health preservation in spring, people should sleep late at night and get up early. In the morning, people can exercise muscles and bones, to keep pleasant moods and avoid getting angry. Because spring is windy, in which people are vulnerable to wind-cold of external contraction, people should exercise to improve body constitution. At the same time, the liver pertains to spring, so liver diseases frequently occur in spring. Anger can hurt the liver, so people should keep pleasant moods and avoid getting angry. Therefore, disease prevention and treatment in TCM are closely related to seasonal climates, the movement of celestial bodies, the sun and moon, which also demonstrates "unity of nature and human." Doctors should also prescribe drugs based on the rules of seasonal change. People in Shanghai tonify body constitution in winter and receive sanfu patch treatment in Chinese dog days of summer, which follow the principle of treatment based on geography and climates.

"Harmony" and "unity of nature and human" are closely related to disease prevention and treatment as well as health preservation. Some people misunderstand health preservation as fear of death. In fact, health preservation is not only for health and longevity, but also for respect for life. According to *The Inner Canon of the Yellow Emperor* (*Huáng Dì Nèi Jīng*, 黄帝内经), health preservation is to defend life, to protect life and to take care of life. There is an article titled "Discourse on Treasuring Life and Preserving Physical Appearance" in *The Inner Canon of the Yellow Emperor* (*Huáng Dì Nèi Jīng*, 黄帝内经). Treasuring life means to cherish life. Preserving physical appearance is to protect the body from being damaged. There is also a very important saying that "nothing in the heaven or on the earth is more miraculous than humanity." That is to say, among all the myriad things in the world, human beings and life are the most noble. *The Divine Pivot* (*Líng Shū*, 灵枢) · *The Jade-Tablets* reads, "between the heaven and the earth, the most precious one is humanity." That is to say, humans are the most precious among all things, which reflect the humanism in *The Inner Canon of the Yellow Emperor* (*Huáng Dì Nèi Jīng*, 黄帝内经). Humanism also involves respect for life. Health preservation is not only for health and longevity, but also for philosophy and culture, that is, respect for life. There is another term about health preservation in *The Inner Canon of the Yellow Emperor* (*Huáng Dì Nèi Jīng*, 黄帝内经), that is "preventive treatment." It would be too late for people to ask for disease prevention and treatment after they are sick. Disease should be prevented before people get sick. Many diseases cannot be cured, such as hypertension, diabetes, coronary heart disease, malignant tumor, etc. Some infectious diseases that endanger human health in the past have been controlled with the development of medicine. However, cardiovascular and cerebrovascular diseases, diabetes mellitus and malignant tumors are all related to behaviors and minds. There is no way to prevent them or take vaccines to control them. People can only rely on health preservation. Why do Chinese people attach so much importance to health preservation? Those diseases that cannot be cured usually require lifelong treatment and medication, which not only make patients suffer, but also increase a lot of medical expenses. Those phenomena show that we should constantly reflect on the purpose of medical treatment. It is necessary to consider why doctors and medical development are so "lagging behind." We should change the idea from treating diseases into preventing diseases. *The Inner Canon of the Yellow Emperor* (*Huáng Dì Nèi Jīng*, 黄帝内经) put forward "preventive treatment" more than 2500 years ago. "Preventive treatment" promotes taking care of health before diseases occur. With the current level of medical treatment, there is no way to completely cure some diseases. The best way is to let yourself not get sick before diseases occur. This is why Chinese people are so keen on health preservation. Health preservation implies a kind of awakening in Chinese people, which is also advocated by Chinese government. We should be alert to potential risks of disease. According to *The Scriptures of Change* (*Yì Jīng*, 易经), "a noble person who is safe does not ignore danger, survives with death in mind, and governs a country without forgetting disorder, so that health can be maintained and the country can be protected." It can be seen from *The Scriptures of Change* (*Yì Jīng*, 易经) and *The Inner Canon of the Yellow Emperor* (*Huáng Dì Nèi Jīng*, 黄帝内经), Chinese people use the same idea to govern the body and govern the country. *The Inner Canon of the Yellow Emperor* (*Huáng Dì Nèi Jīng*, 黄帝内经) reads that "disease should be prevented before it occurs, and disorder should be avoided before it happens." A country should manage affairs before it is in chaos, otherwise it would be too late. Therefore, leaders often remind us of being alert to potential risks, and human body also needs to be alert to potential risks of disease. When there is no disease, people need to take precautions, especially after the age of 40. *The Inner Canon of the Yellow Emperor* (*Huáng Dì Nèi Jīng*, 黄帝内经) reads that "at the age of 40, yin Qi is reduced to half." That is to say, after 40 years old, people begin to get old and feeble; women will have crow's feet; men will have gray temples, with kidney qi getting gradually deficient. Therefore, health preservation is about investment in health, which is very important. When the body gets old, diseases could occur. Usually, from 50 to 60 years old is a peak period of illness. In short, health preservation should start from the time when there is no disease and when you are young. It is too late to start when you are sick. *Masters from Huainan* (*Huái Nán Zǐ*, 淮南子) reads that "good doctors prevent disease and sages avoid troubles." A good doctor governs the body and a good minister governs the country. Both the country and the body should be alert to potential risks.

Sun Simiao, born in Tang dynasty, was an expert of health preservation and medicine in Chinese history. Studies showed that the life span of people in Tang dynasty was about 33 years old, while Sun Simiao lived to 140 years old. He said that "best doctors prevent disease; moderate doctors intervene when disease is about to occur; mediocre doctors treat diseases." He divided people into three categories. One category is in good health without disease. The second category is in sub-health with occasional poor sleep, poor appetite, constipation, fatigue, whose physical and chemical examination results are normal or at the boundary. The third category is being sick. Doctors can also be divided into three categories, including the best doctors, moderate doctors and mediocre doctors. The best doctors protect people from getting sick, through health preservation. Moderate doctors help people who are about to get sick restore health. Mediocre doctors treat diseases. We all hope that we are the best doctors and share methods of health preservation in *The Inner Canon of the Yellow Emperor* (*Huáng Dì Nèi Jīng*, 黄帝内经) with more people. It was extraordinary that people in Tang dynasty had the thought of health preservation, which is still fully in line with the national conditions of China.

10.5 Personal views on health preservation

(1) HEALTH PRESERVATION AT THE RIGHT TIME BASED ON "UNITY OF NATURE AND HUMAN"

What is the meaning of health preservation at the right time? To put it simply, we should arrange our daily lives, including spiritual activities, according to the four seasons. That is to say, we should live regularly. In today's society, many people are against the law of nature to arrange eating and living. For example, some people stay up late to work, to play games or sing karaoke for entertainment until midnight. A day and night is divided into 12 two-hour periods, which involves a process of waxing and waning of yin and yang. Many people fail to eat regularly, sleep regularly, work or live regularly, which is the ultimate cause of sub-health and many diseases. It doesn't really matter if unhealthy lifestyle lasts one or two months. If it lasts too long, the biological clock will be disordered, causing dysfunction, which gives chances to viruses, bacteria and other pathogenic factors to attack human body. For example, physiological dysfunction can be manifested at first, followed by organic disease, then organ failure, and finally death. People can try to identify which phase they are in? Is it a phase of not being sick, almost getting sick or already getting sick? The first requirement of health preservation is to live regularly according to time and seasons.

(2) MENTAL HEALTH PRESERVATION BASED ON TAOIST "SIMPLE LIVING AND PEACE"

To preserve health firstly requires to cultivate minds. How can one cultivate minds? This topic is involved in *The Inner Canon of the Yellow Emperor* (*Huáng Dì Nèi Jīng*, 黄帝内经) and other literatures in past generations. I once wrote *Dictionary of Famous Articles on Health Preservation of Chinese Medicine* (*Guó Yī Yǎng Shēng Míng Piān Jiàn Shǎng Cí Diǎn*, 国医养生名篇鉴赏辞典), which collected the contents of health preservation in medical literatures from the Spring and Autumn period and the Warring States period to modern times, including the contents in *The Analects of Confucius* (*Lún Yǔ*, 论语) and *Tao Te Ching* (*Dào Dé Jīng*, 道德经), as well as some famous works unrelated to medicine in the past dynasties. That book attracted large numbers of readers. An important idea in the book is that simple living and peace are critical in health preservation. Zhuge Liang said that "simple living show high ideals; slow and steady wins the race." It is not easy for people to achieve that, because they need to control desires. Desire is a double-edged sword. If there is a desire, there will be a demand which can push people work hard and make the society progress. However, once desires go beyond individuals' ability to bear, they will become pathogenic factors. Many diseases are caused by uncontrolled desires. Therefore, traditional Chinese culture, and medical works such as *The Inner Canon of the Yellow Emperor* (*Huáng Dì Nèi Jīng*, 黄帝内经), put emphasizes on controlling desire and maintaining simple living and peace. To live a simple life requires peace, and the peace refers to the peace of mind. We should adjust desires. Humans are self-contradictory. If a desire is not satisfied, they will suffer, and if all the desires are satisfied, they will be bored. So, it is difficult to balance. In clinical practice, some patients came to me, complaining of insomnia, fatigue, poor appetite, with normal results of physical examination. They said that they were not happy although they have houses and cars, lack of nothing. That is because they lack spiritual sustenance. Therefore, mental health care is even more important than physical health preservation.

(3) HEALTHY DIET BASED ON "HARMONY OF TASTES"

The Inner Canon of the Yellow Emperor (*Huáng Dì Nèi Jīng*, 黄帝内经) put forward the concept of "diet with restraint." The restraint here has two meanings. One is to control diet, and the other is to have regular diets. Some people eat food during 1 a.m. to 2 a.m. after staying up late to play games, sing karaoke, or work. But intestines and stomach need rest at midnight. Some people even go to sleep immediately after eating, and then something goes wrong. With high blood cholesterol, increased blood viscosity, and clogged arteries, eating greasy food at midnight may block blood vessels all of a sudden. The next morning such patients cannot get up, and they can have angina, cerebral infarction, and myocardial infarction, which are frequently seen cases in clinical practice. Therefore, harmony of tastes is to maintain a reasonable diet with balanced nutrition, which is also advocated by the World Health Organization.

(4) EXERCISE FOR HEALTH PRESERVATION BASED ON "MOVEMENT WITH RESTRAINT"

Life lies in movement, but traditional Chinese medicine believes that people should move with restraint. If someone has myocardial ischemia, or hemangioma, vigorous exercise can make them die faster. Strenuous exercises such as climbing mountains and stairs will accelerate the occurrence of osteoarthritis among the elderly with osteoporosis. Therefore, it is necessary to exercise in a moderate way. An important principle in sports is to stop when necessary. *The Inner Canon of the Yellow Emperor: Basic Questions* (*Huáng Dì Nèi Jīng Sù Wèn*, 黄帝内经素问) reads "proper exertion," which means that people should work and move when alive, benefiting the circulation of Qi and blood. But it is not to make the body too tired. Many people have chronic fatigue syndrome, especially people in sub-health, who do not follow the principle of "movement with restraint." No matter it is for physical exercise or mental exercise, "movement with restraint" should be obeyed. Therefore, the thoughts in *The Inner Canon of the Yellow Emperor* (*Huáng Dì Nèi Jīng*, 黄帝内经) are actually very profound.

(5) "BENEVOLENCE COMES WITH LONGEVITY"

The World Health Organization mentioned moral health in the definition of health. TCM also puts emphasis on it long time ago. Confucius proposed that "benevolence comes with longevity" and "great virtues contributes to longevity." A moral person with benevolence tends to live longer. From the perspective of psychosomatic medicine, a moral person must be healthy and postive mentally. It was found that the elderly over 100 years old in Shanghai had one thing in common. They are kind-hearted with benevolence, who have harmonious families, and harmonious relationships with neighborhood, and whose children have filial piety. When they were working, the relationships between them and colleagues were very good. Those people are positive, and in terms of psychology, they are mentally healthy. They do not get entangled in trifles. Ji Xianlin lived until he was 98 years old. He has three principles of health preservation. The first is to eat less; the second is not to move; the third is to be good-tempered. Therefore, benevolence benefits mental health.

10.6 Some comments about health

Firstly, some healthy people often does not preserve health. They plan to keep fit after getting old or after retirement. But as mentioned before it, it would be too late then.

Secondly, silly people often abuse health. Some people pursue careers, but ignore health. They often overuse health for the sake of careers to have organic diseases. Professor Yu Juan in Fudan University studied for a master's degree and then a doctor's degree. She was promoted to an associate professor and then to a full professor. After she got cancer, she wrote a book to tell people to control desires, and not to overuse health for fame and wealth. But it was too late for her to repent, so we should learn from her experience.

Thirdly, people should learn to save health. To save money, we deposit money in the bank. In fact, health also needs to be saved. *The Inner Canon of the Yellow Emperor* (*Huáng Dì Nèi Jīng*, 黄帝内经) explains that after 40 years old, health begins to decline, and people should reserve health to prevent disease.

Fourthly, wise people should actively invest in health. To invest in health does not mean buying lots of Xiyangshen (西洋参, Radix Panacis Quinquefolii), Dongchongxiacao (冬虫夏草, Cordyceps) and other supplements. The investment means that we should arrange our life scientifically, reasonably and properly for health preservation. "Without health, there will be no well-off society." The premise of a well-off society is healthy citizens with good mental health. Without health, no one can enjoy a better life.

At last, life is actually a natural phenomenon. Health and longevity also have its own limits. You cannot live as long as you want. Many emperors in history looked for the elixir of immortality, but there is no such elixir in the world. According to statistics, there were more than 480 emperors in Chinese feudal society, among which only a dozen of them lived to 80 years old. Most of them were short-lived. Now the life expectancy of people in Shanghai is more than 82 years old, and the average life expectancy of Chinese people is more than 76 years old. What does that mean? With the improvement of living standards, health awareness and health standards, people become active to preserve health. Therefore, people do not need to pursue health and longevity on purpose, but the value and significance of life. Qian Xuesen lived to be 98, and Ji Xianlin lived to be 98. They were busy working with enterprise, who also made great achievements. They were not waiting there to become 98 years old. They lived for pursuits and careers. Therefore, it is the best to preserve health in the pursuit of life value at the same time. We should face life calmly, be happy and enjoy life, and experience the reality. Only in this way can we have a harmonious life and live a long and healthy life.

In short, health preservation is to develop a healthy lifestyle. Let's do it together!

ABOUT THE AUTHOR

ZHU HUIRONG, female, research professor and doctoral supervisor. Her research focuses on the prevention and treatment of malignant tumors with traditional Chinese medicine.

Currently, she is the Deputy Secretary of the Party Committee and Vice President of Shanghai University of Traditional Chinese Medicine. She concurrently serves as the deputy chairman of the Collateral Disease Branch, Chinese Association of Chinese Medicine, the chairman of the Collateral Disease Branch, Shanghai Association of Chinese Medicine, the chairman of the Ethics Committee, Shanghai Association of Chinese Integrative Medicine, and the deputy chairman of the Oncology Branch, Shanghai Association of Chinese Medicine.

In addition, she has been dedicated to psychological theories and practices from the perspective of traditional Chinese medicine. She is undertaking the moral education theoretic research project of universities in Shanghai, namely the *"Research on the Construction of the Localization Mode of College Students' Psychological Health Education from the Perspective of Chinese Medicine Culture."* She has also edited *"MIND HEALING – Ten Lectures by TCM Experts"* and published over 50 academic papers in the past five years.